What's New in This Edition?

Twenty-five years ago we self-published our first version of *Stretching*. Five years later, in 1980, we teamed up with Shelter Publications to produce a revised version of *Stretching* for bookstores. Since then the book has gone on to become an international best-seller.

Now, some 20 years later, we've decided to do a new revision of *Stretching*. Here's what's different in this edition:

• All of the drawings are new.

• There are are 11 new everyday routines:

   Hands, Arms, and Shoulders • Neck, Shoulders, and Arms • Legs, Groin, and Hips • Lower Back Tension • After Sitting • Computer and Desk Stretches • Blue-Collar Stretches • Stretches for Kids • Gardening Stretches • Airplane Stretches • Traveler's Stretches

• There are 14 new sports routines:

   Aerobic Exercise • Badminton • Bowling • Equestrian Sports • Inline Skating • Kayaking • Motocross • Mountain Biking • Rock Climbing • Rodeo • Snowboarding • Table Tennis • Triathlon • Windsurfing

• In the stretching routines, both men and women are shown doing the stretches, and are wearing the clothing of their sport or activity.

• For people in a hurry, each sport routine has a mini-routine.

• Warming up before stretching is recommended for the more vigorous activities to avoid possible injuries.

• Certain of the more difficult stretches have been eliminated.

• Times for holding some stretches have been reduced.

• There is a new section on PNF stretching, a more complex, but easily learned technique for increasing flexibility. *(See pp. 206–209.)*

• There is a section on body tools, which can be very effective, especially when used with stretching.

We hope you like this new book, and that it helps you remain limber and in good health for the rest of your life!

—Bob and Jean Anderson

STRETCHING

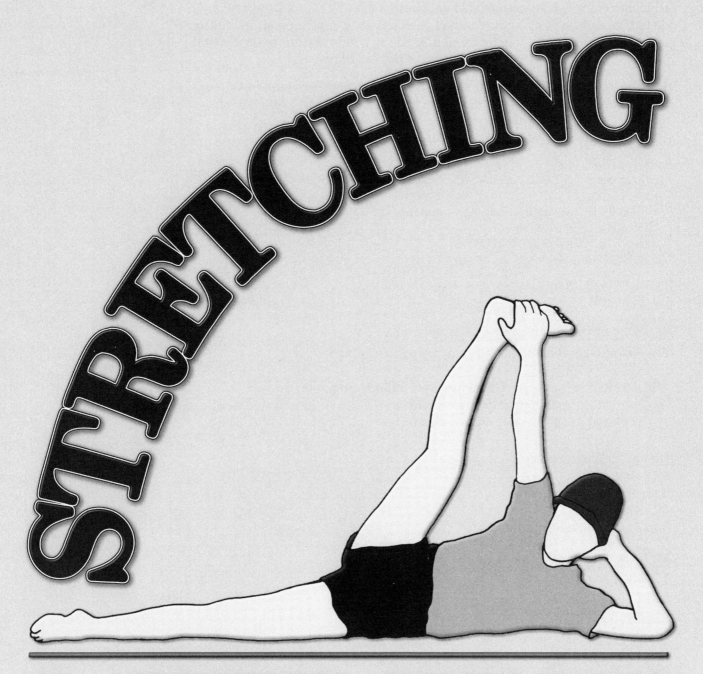

20TH ANNIVERSARY · REVISED EDITION

BOB ANDERSON

Illustrated by JEAN ANDERSON

Distributed in the United States by Publishers Group West and in Canada by Publishers Group Canada

Library of Congress Cataloging-in-Publication Data

Anderson, Bob, 1945–
    Stretching / by Bob Anderson ; illustrated by Jean Anderson — Rev. ed.
       p.   cm.
    Includes bibliographical references and index.
    ISBN-10: 0-936070-22-6
    ISBN-13: 978-0-936070-22-3
    1. Stretching exercises   I. Title

RA781.63 .A527 2000
613.7'1 — dc21   00-036525

14 13 12 — 12 11 10 09
(Lowest digits indicate number and year of latest printing.)

 Printed on acid-free Glatfelter Thor Plus D-56 paper, with 15% post-consumer waste content
Printed in the United States of America

Shelter Publications, Inc.
P. O. Box 279
Bolinas, California 94924
415-868-0280
Email: shelter@shelterpub.com

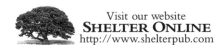
Visit our website
SHELTER ONLINE
http://www.shelterpub.com

Contents

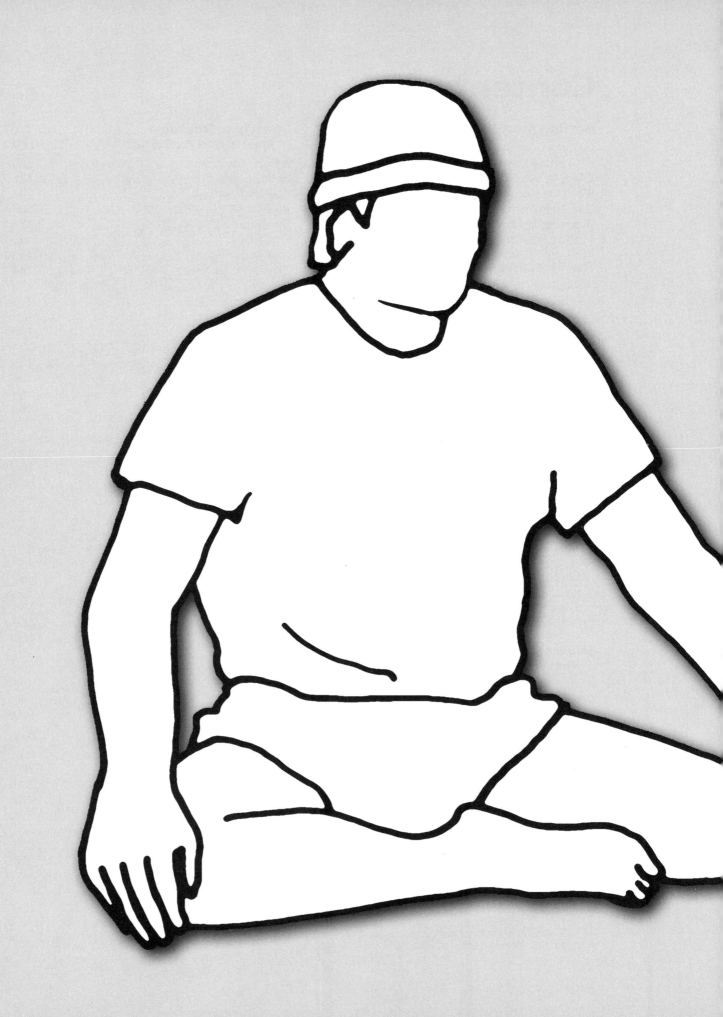

GETTING STARTED

This first section is an introduction to stretching. It is very important to read pages 12–13, "How to Stretch," so you will understand how to do the stretches in the rest of the book. Then, if you are new to stretching, the section "Getting Started," on pages 15–21, will take you through a series of simple stretches.

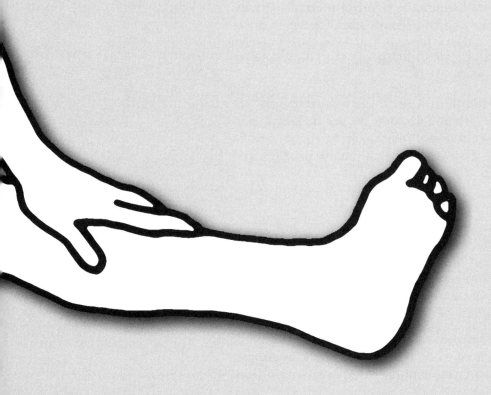

Introduction

Today millions of people have discovered the benefits of movement. Everywhere you look they are out, running, cycling, skating, playing tennis, or swimming. What do they hope to accomplish? Why this relatively sudden interest in physical fitness?

Many recent studies have shown that active people lead fuller lives. They have more stamina, resist illness, and stay trim. They have more self-confidence, are less depressed, and often, even late in life, are still working energetically on new projects.

Medical research has shown that a great deal of ill health is directly related to lack of physical activity. Awareness of this fact, along with fuller knowledge of health care, is changing lifestyles. The current enthusiasm for movement is not a fad. We now realize that the only way to prevent the diseases of inactivity is to remain active—not for a month, or a year, but for a lifetime.

* * * *

Our ancestors did not have the problems that go with a sedentary life; they had to work hard to survive. They stayed strong and healthy through continuous, vigorous outdoor work: chopping, digging, tilling, planting, hunting, and all their other daily activities. But with the advent of the Industrial Revolution, machines began to do the work once done by hand. As people became less active, they began to lose strength and the instinct for natural movement.

Machines have obviously made life easier, but they have also created serious problems. Instead of walking, we drive; rather than climb stairs, we use elevators; while once we were almost continuously active, we now spend much of our lives sitting. Computers have made us even more sedentary. Without daily physical exertion, our bodies become storehouses of unreleased tensions. With no natural outlets for our tensions, our muscles become weak and tight, and we lose touch with our physical nature, with life's energies.

But times have changed. We have found that health is something we can control, that we can prevent poor health and disease. We are no longer content to sit and stagnate. Now we are moving, rediscovering the joys of an active, healthy life. What's more, we can resume a more healthy and rewarding existence at any age.

* * * *

The body's capacity for recovery is phenomenal. For example, a surgeon makes an incision, removes or corrects the problem, then sews you back up. At this point, the body takes over and heals itself. Nature finishes the surgeon's job. All of us have this seemingly miraculous capacity for regaining health, whether it's from something as drastic as surgery, or from poor physical condition caused by lack of activity and bad diet.

What does stretching have to do with all this? It is the important link between the sedentary life and the active life. It keeps the muscles supple, prepares you for movement, and helps you make the daily transition from inactivity to vigorous activity without undue strain. It is especially important if you run, cycle, play tennis, or engage in other strenuous exercises, because activities like these promote tightness and inflexibility. Stretching before and after you work out will keep you flexible and may prevent common injuries such as knee problems from running and sore shoulders or elbows from tennis.

With the tremendous number of people exercising now, the need for correct information is vital. Stretching is easy, but when it is done incorrectly, it can actually do more harm than good. For this reason it is essential to understand the right techniques.

* * * *

Over the past three decades I have worked with amateur and professional athletic teams and have participated in various sports medicine clinics throughout the country. I have been able to teach athletes that stretching is a simple, painless way of getting ready for movement. They have found it enjoyable and easy to do. And when they have stretched regularly and correctly, it has helped them avoid injuries and perform to the best of their abilities.

Stretching feels good when done correctly. You do not have to push limits or attempt to go further each day. It should not be a personal contest to see how far you can stretch. Stretching should be tailored to your particular muscular structure, flexibility, and varying tension levels. The key is regularity and relaxation. The object is to reduce muscular tension, thereby promoting freer movement—not to concentrate on attaining extreme flexibility, which often leads to overstretching and injury.

We can learn a lot by observing animals. Watch a cat. It instinctively knows how to stretch. It does so spontaneously, never overstretching, continually and naturally tuning up muscles it will have to use.

* * * *

Stretching is not stressful. It is peaceful, relaxing, and noncompetitive. The subtle, invigorating feelings of stretching allow you to get in touch with your muscles. It is completely adjustable to the individual. You do not have to conform to any unyielding discipline; stretching gives you the freedom to be yourself and enjoy being yourself.

Anyone can be fit, with the right approach. You don't need to be a great athlete. But you do need to take it slowly, especially in the beginning. Give your body and mind time to adjust to the stresses of physical activity. Start easily and be regular. There is no way to get into shape in a day.

When you are stretching regularly and exercising frequently, you will learn to enjoy movement. Remember that each one of us is a unique physical and mental being with our own comfortable and enjoyable rhythms. We are all different in strength, endurance, flexibility, and temperament. If you learn about your body and its needs, you will be able to develop your own personal potential and gradually build a foundation of fitness that will last a lifetime.

Who Should Stretch

Everyone can learn to stretch, regardless of age or flexibility. You do not need to be in top physical condition or have specific athletic skills. Whether you sit at a desk all day, dig ditches, do housework, stand at an assembly line, drive a truck, or exercise regularly, the same techniques of stretching apply. The methods are gentle and easy, conforming to individual differences in muscle tension and flexibility. So, if you are healthy, without any specific physical problems, you can learn how to stretch safely and enjoyably.

> **Note:** If you have had any recent physical problems or surgery, particularly of the joints and muscles, or if you have been inactive or sedentary for some time, please consult your professional health care professional before you start a stretching or exercise program.

When to Stretch

Stretching can be done any time you feel like it: at work, in a car, waiting for a bus, walking down the road, under a nice shady tree after a hike, or at the beach. Stretch before and after physical activity, but also stretch at various times of the day when you can. Here are some examples:

- In the morning before the start of the day.
- At work to release nervous tension.
- After sitting or standing for a long time.
- When you feel stiff.
- At odd times during the day, as for instance, when watching TV, listening to music, reading, or sitting and talking.

Why Stretch

Stretching, because it relaxes your mind and tunes up your body, should be part of your daily life. You will find that regular stretching will do the following things:

- Reduce muscle tension and make the body feel more relaxed
- Help coordination by allowing for freer and easier movement
- Increase range of motion
- Help prevent injuries such as muscle strains. (A strong, flexible, pre-stretched muscle resists stress better than a strong, stiff, unstretched muscle.)
- Make strenuous activities like running, skiing, tennis, swimming, and cycling easier because it prepares you for activity; it's a way of signaling the muscles that they are about to be used.
- Helps maintain your current level of flexibility, so as time passes you do not become stiffer and stiffer
- Develop body awareness; as you stretch various parts of the body, you focus on them and get in touch with them; you get to know yourself.
- Help loosen the mind's control of the body so that the body moves for "its own sake" rather than for competition or ego
- Feel good

How to Stretch

Stretching is easy to learn. But there is a right way and a wrong way to stretch. The right way is a relaxed, sustained stretch with your attention focused on the muscles being stretched. The wrong way (unfortunately practiced by many people) is to bounce up and down or to stretch to the point of pain: these methods can actually do more harm than good.

If you stretch correctly and regularly, you will find that every movement you make becomes easier. It will take time to loosen up tight muscles or muscle groups, but time is quickly forgotten when you start to feel good.

The Easy Stretch

When you begin a stretch, spend 10–15 seconds in the *easy stretch*. No bouncing! Go to the point where you feel a *mild tension,* and relax as you hold the stretch. The feeling of tension should subside as you hold the position. If it does not, ease off slightly and find a degree of tension that is comfortable. You should be able to say, "I feel the stretch, but it is not painful." The easy stretch reduces muscular tightness and tension and readies the tissues for the developmental stretch.

The Developmental Stretch

After the easy stretch, move slowly into the *developmental stretch*. Again, no bouncing. Move a fraction of an inch further until you again feel a mild tension and hold for 10–15 seconds. Be in control. Again, the tension should diminish; if not, ease off slightly. Remember: If the stretch tension increases as the stretch is held and/or it becomes painful, you are stretching too far! The developmental stretch fine-tunes the muscles and increases flexibility.

Breathing

Your breathing should be slow, rhythmical, and under control. If you are bending forward to do a stretch, exhale as you bend forward and then breathe slowly as you hold the stretch. Do not hold your breath while stretching. If a stretch position inhibits your natural breathing pattern, then you are obviously not relaxed. Just ease up on the stretch so you can breathe naturally.

Counting

At first, silently count the seconds for each stretch; this will insure that you hold the proper tension for a long enough time. After a while, you will be stretching by the way it feels, without the distraction of counting.

The Stretch Reflex

Your muscles are protected by a mechanism called the *stretch reflex*. Any time you stretch the muscle fibers too far (either by bouncing or over-stretching), a nerve reflex responds by sending a signal to the muscles to contract; this keeps the muscles from being injured. Thus, stretching too far tightens the very muscles you are trying to stretch! (You get a similar involuntary muscle reaction when you accidentally touch something hot; before you can think about it, your body jerks away from the heat.)

Pushing a stretch too far or bouncing up and down strains the muscles and activates the stretch reflex. This causes pain, as well as physical damage due to the microscopic tearing of muscle fibers. This in turn leads to the formation of scar tissue in the muscles, with a gradual loss of elasticity. The muscles become stiff and sore. It's hard to get enthused about daily stretching and exercise when you're pushing it to the point of pain!

No Gain *with* Pain

Many of us were conditioned in high school to the idea of "no gain without pain." We learned to associate pain with physical improvement, and were taught that "... the more it hurts, the more you get out of it." Don't be fooled. Stretching, when done correctly, is not painful. Learn to pay attention to your body, for pain is an indication that something is *wrong*.

The easy and developmental stretches, as described on the previous page, do not overactivate the stretch reflex and do not cause pain.

This Diagram Will Give You an Idea of a "Good Stretch"

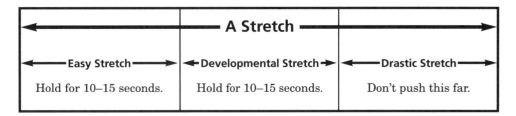

The straight-line diagram represents the stretch that is possible with your muscles and their connective tissue. You will find that your flexibility will naturally increase when you stretch, first in the easy, then in the developmental phase. By stretching regularly and staying relaxed, you will be able to go beyond your present limits and come closer to your personal potential.

Warming Up and Cooling Down

Warming Up

There has been some controversy in recent years about stretching before you warm up. If you are going to stretch, will you get injured if you stretch without specifically warming up first? No—if you stretch comfortably and not strenuously. However, I suggest that you do several minutes of general movement (walking and swinging arms, etc.) to warm the muscles and related soft tissue before you stretch. This will get the blood moving. You still have to stretch correctly whether you are warmed up or not.

Some runners have reported they are more likely to get injured if they don't warm up before stretching. It is possible to get hurt stretching if:

• you are in too much of a hurry (not relaxed)
• you push too far, too soon (overstretching a cold muscle)
• you are not paying attention to the feeling of the stretch

You will not get hurt stretching if you stretch correctly *(see pp.12–13)*. You will sense how far to stretch if you are paying attention to how the stretch feels; tune into your body.

Here's my advice if you are engaging in an activity such as running or cycling or whatever: Warm up by doing the activity you are about to do, but at a lower intensity. For example, if you are about to run—walk or jog for 2–5 minutes or until you break a light sweat. (Walking and jogging provide a good, basic warm-up for many activities. This will increase muscle and blood temperature and raise total body temperature to provide an effective warm-up.) Then stretch.

Cooling Down

Conversely, you should cool down after exercise by doing a scaled-down version of the main workout. Get your heart rate back down towards a resting rate. Then stretch to prevent muscle soreness and stiffness.

Getting Started

Here we will walk you through nine stretches that will help you to understand the phrase "Go with the *feel* of the stretch." Once you understand this technique, it will be easy to learn and use the stretches in this book.

Note: Dotted areas indicate the parts of the body in which you will probably feel the stretch, but because no two people are the same, it is possible that you may feel a stretch in an area other than those marked.

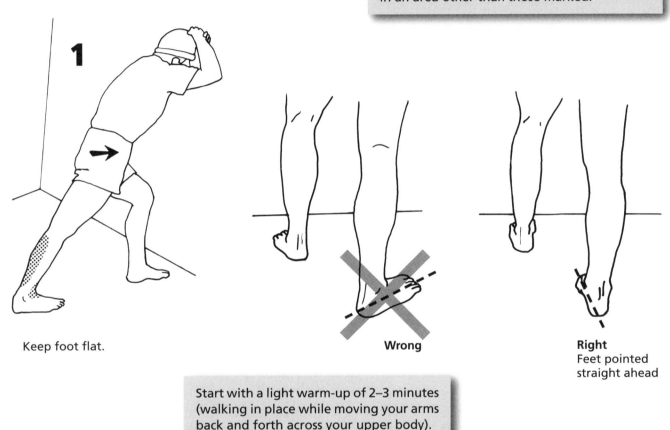

Keep foot flat.

Wrong

Right
Feet pointed
straight ahead

Start with a light warm-up of 2–3 minutes (walking in place while moving your arms back and forth across your upper body).

First we'll do a calf stretch. Lean on your forearms, using a wall, or something else for support. Rest your forehead on the back of your hands. Bend one knee and bring it toward the support. The back leg should be straight, with the foot flat and pointed straight ahead or slightly toed-in.

Now, without changing the position of your feet, slowly move your hips forward as you keep the back leg straight and your *foot flat*. Create an *easy feeling* of stretch in your calf muscle.

Hold an easy stretch for 10 seconds, then move slightly further into a developmental stretch for 10 seconds. Don't overstretch.

Now stretch the other calf. Does one leg feel different from the other? Is one leg more flexible than the other?

Sitting Groin Stretch: Next, sit on the floor. Clasp the soles of your feet together with your hands as shown. Gently lean forward *from the hips* until you feel an easy stretch in your groin. Contract your abdominal muscles mildly as you go into the stretch. Hold an easy stretch for 15 seconds. If you are doing it right, it will feel good; the longer you hold the stretch, the less you should feel it. If possible, without strain, keep your elbows on the outside of your lower legs. This will help give you stability and balance.

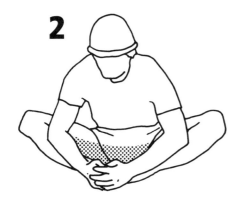

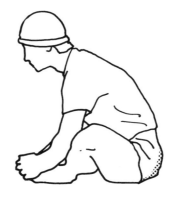

Exhale as you go into the stretch. Breathe slowly and rhythmically as you hold it. Relax your jaw and shoulders.

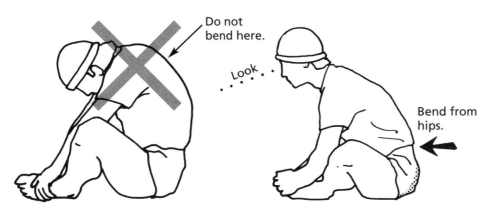

Do not bend here.

Look

Bend from hips.

Do not bend forward from your head and shoulders. This rounds the shoulders and puts pressure on lower back.

Concentrate on making the initial move forward from your hips. Keep your lower back flat. Look out in front of you.

After you feel the tension diminish slightly, increase the stretch by gently pulling yourself a little further into the stretch feeling. Now it should feel a bit more intense *but not painful.* Hold for about 15 seconds. The feeling of tension should decrease slightly the longer the stretch is held. Slowly come out of the stretch. Please, no jerky, quick, bouncing movements!

Stretch by the *feel* of the stretch, not by how *far* you can stretch.

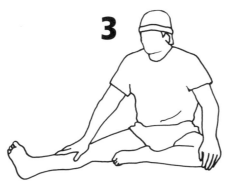

3

Next, straighten the right leg as you keep the left leg bent. The sole of the left foot should be facing the inside of the right upper leg. Do not keep the knee of the straight leg "locked." You are in a straight-leg, bent-knee position.

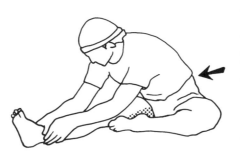

Now, to stretch the hamstrings and left side of the lower back (some will feel a stretch in the lower back, others won't), bend forward *from your hips* as you exhale until you feel a very slight stretch. Hold for 10–15 seconds. Breathe slowly and rhythmically. Touch the quadriceps of your right thigh to make sure that these muscles are relaxed. They should be soft, not tight.

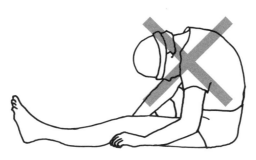

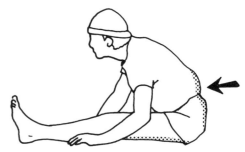

Don't make the initial movement with your head and shoulders. Don't try to touch your forehead to your knee. This will only round your shoulders.

Do initiate the stretch from the hips. Keep your chin in a neutral position. Keep your shoulders and arms relaxed.

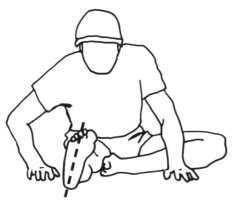

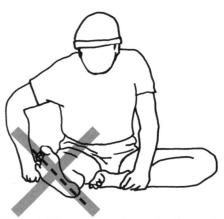

Be sure the foot of the leg being stretched is upright, with the ankle and toes relaxed. This will keep you aligned through the ankle, knee, and hip.

Do not let your leg turn to the outside because this causes misalignment of the leg and hip.

If you are not very flexible, use a towel around the bottom of your foot to do this stretch.

After the feeling of the easy stretch has subsided, slowly go into the developmental stretch for 10–15 seconds. You may only have to bend forward a fraction of an inch. Do not worry about how far you can go. Remember, we are all different.

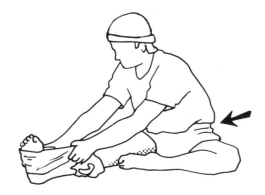

Slowly come out of the stretch. Do the same stretch on the other side. Keep the front of your thigh relaxed and your foot upright, with ankle and toes relaxed. Do an easy stretch for 15 seconds, and then slowly find the developmental phase of the stretch and hold for 10–15 seconds.

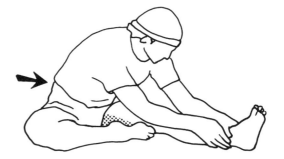

It takes time and sensitivity to stretch properly.

Develop your ability to stretch by how you feel and not by how far you can stretch.

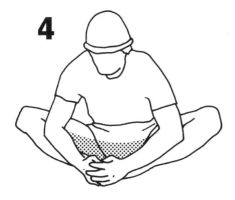

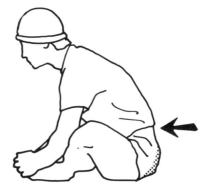

Repeat the sitting groin stretch. How does this feel as compared to the first time you did it? Any change at all?

A number of things are more important than concentrating solely on increasing flexibility:

1. Relaxation of tense areas such as feet, hands, wrists, shoulders, and jaw when stretching
2. Learning how to find and control the right amount of tension in each stretch
3. Awareness of lower back, head and shoulders, and leg alignment during the stretch
4. Adjusting to daily changes, for every day the body feels slightly different

5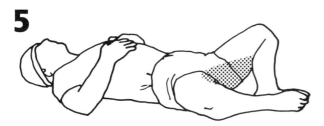

Lying Groin Stretch: Now lie on your back with the soles of your feet together. Let your knees fall apart. Relax your hips and let gravity give you a very mild stretch in your groin. Stay in this very relaxed position for 40 seconds. Breathe deeply.

Let go of any tension. The stretch feeling here will be subtle.

6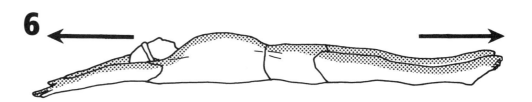

Elongation Stretch: Slowly straighten both legs. With your arms overhead, reach out with your hands while pointing your toes. Hold for 5 seconds, then relax. Repeat 3 times. Each time you stretch, gently pull in your abdominal muscles to make the middle of your body thin. This feels really good. It stretches arms, shoulders, spine, abdominals, as well as muscles of the rib cage, feet, and ankles. This is a great stretch to do first thing in the morning while still in bed.

7

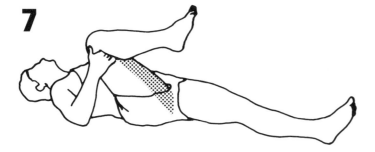

Next, bend one knee and gently pull it toward your chest until you feel an easy stretch. Hold for 30 seconds. You may feel a stretch in your lower back and back of the upper leg. If you do not feel any stretch, don't worry about it. This is an excellent position for the entire body, good for the lower back and very relaxing whether you feel a stretch or not. Do both sides and compare. Do not hold your breath.

Gradually get to know yourself.

8

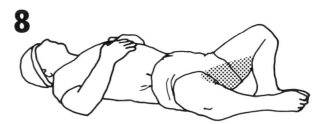

Repeat the lying groin stretch and relax for 30 seconds. Let go of any tension in your feet, hands, and shoulders. You may want to do this stretch with your eyes closed.

How to Sit Up from a Lying Position

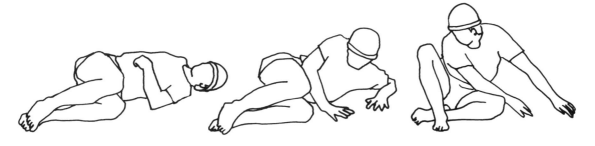

Bend both knees and roll over onto one side. While resting on your side, use your hands to push yourself up into a sitting position. By using your hands and arms this way, you take the pressure or stress off the back.

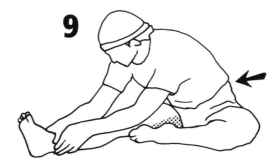

9 Now repeat the stretches for your hamstrings. Have you changed at all? Do you feel more limber and less tense than before stretching?

SUMMARY

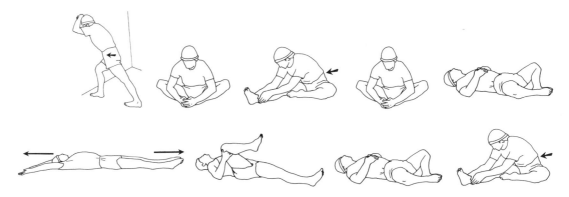

These are just a few stretches to get you started. I want you to understand that stretching is not a contest in flexibility. Your flexibility will naturally improve with proper stretching. Stretch with feelings you can enjoy.

Many of the stretches should be held for 20–30 seconds. But after a while the time you hold stretches will vary. Sometimes you may want to hold a stretch longer because you are extra tight that day, or you are just enjoying the stretch. Or you may not want to hold a stretch as long when your body already feels fairly limber; this would generally be when you hold a stretch for 5–15 seconds. *Remember that no two days are the same* so you must gauge your stretching by how you feel at the moment.

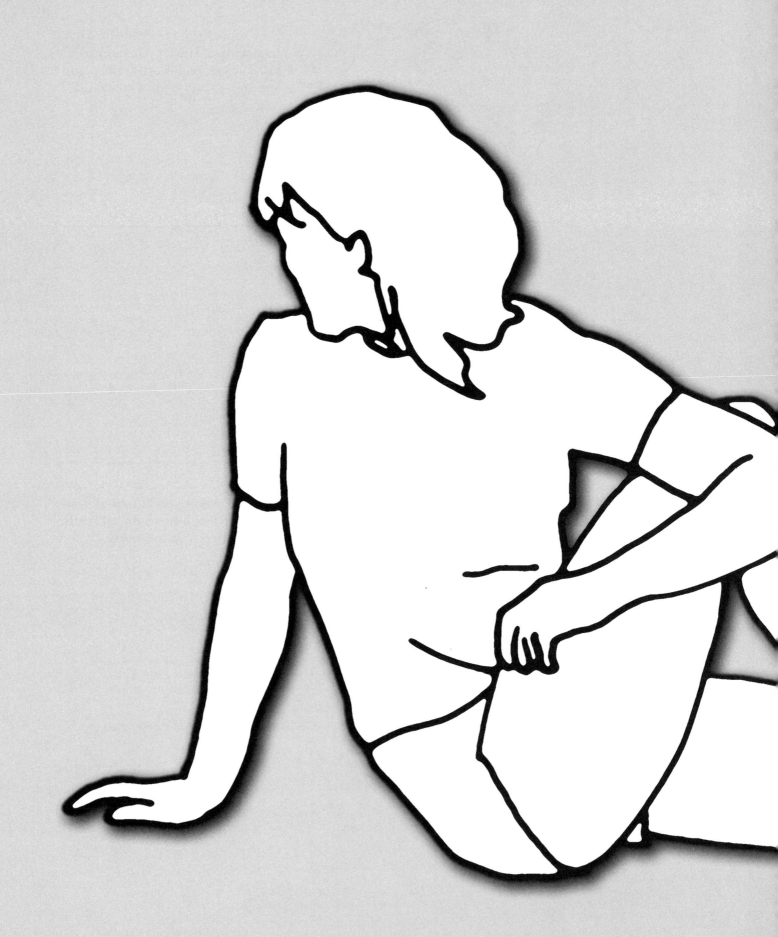

THE STRETCHES

In the following section *(pp. 26–103)* are all the stretches in the book, with instructions for each position. They are grouped according to body parts and presented as a series, but any of them may be done separately without doing the entire routine.

Note: You need not stretch as far as the drawings indicate. Stretch by how you feel without trying to imitate the figure in the drawings. Adjust each stretch to your own personal flexibility, which will vary daily.

Learn stretches for the various parts of the body, at first concentrating on the areas of greatest tension or tightness. On the next two pages is a guide to various muscles and body parts, with reference to the page where each may be found in the book.

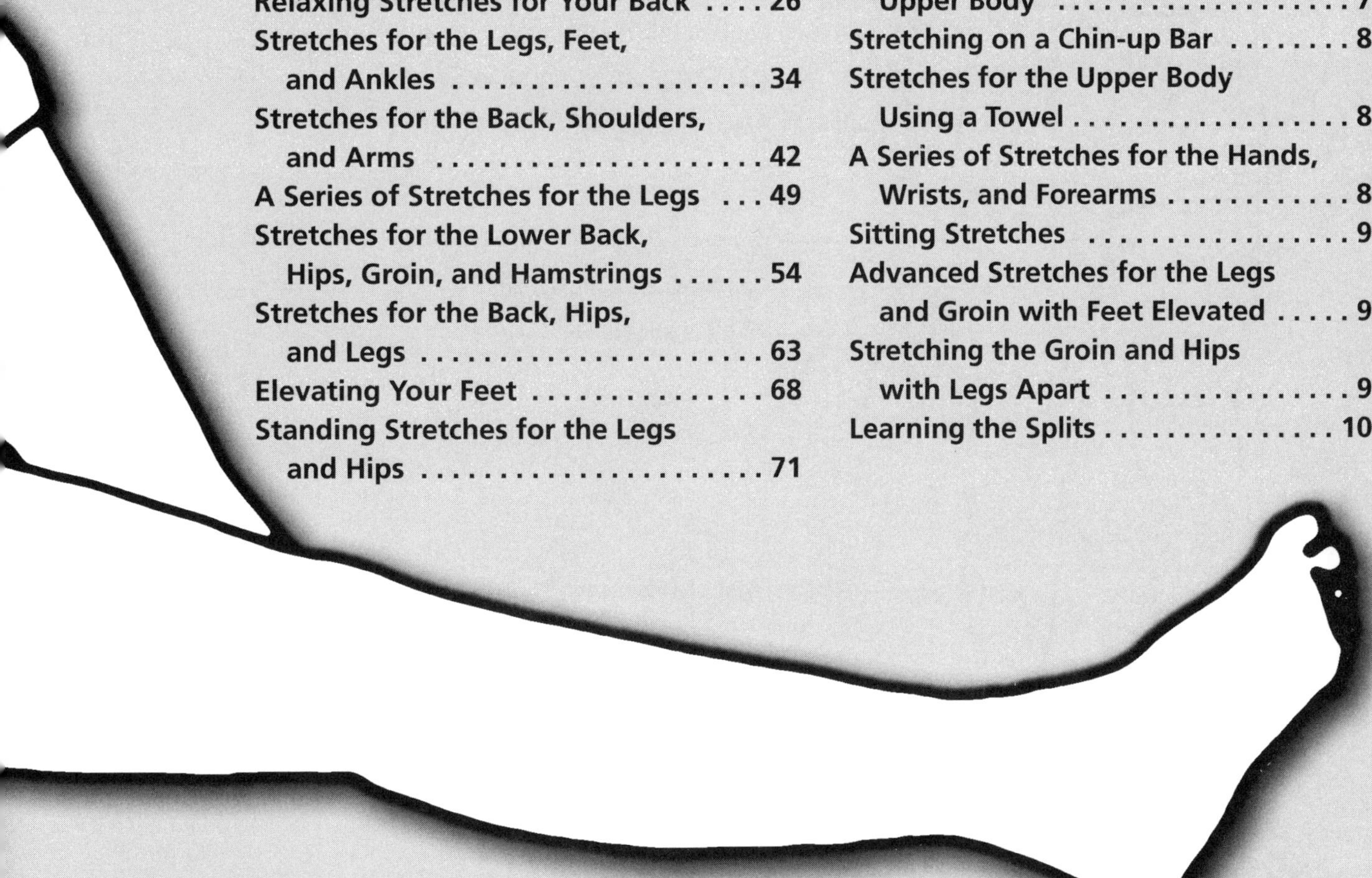

Stretching Guide

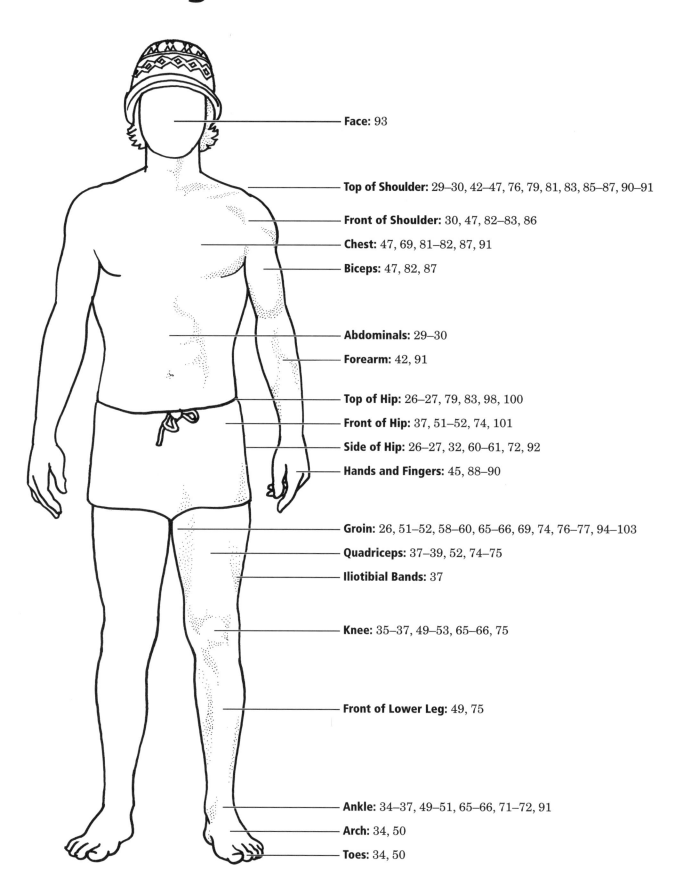

Face: 93

Top of Shoulder: 29–30, 42–47, 76, 79, 81, 83, 85–87, 90–91

Front of Shoulder: 30, 47, 82–83, 86

Chest: 47, 69, 81–82, 87, 91

Biceps: 47, 82, 87

Abdominals: 29–30

Forearm: 42, 91

Top of Hip: 26–27, 79, 83, 98, 100

Front of Hip: 37, 51–52, 74, 101

Side of Hip: 26–27, 32, 60–61, 72, 92

Hands and Fingers: 45, 88–90

Groin: 26, 51–52, 58–60, 65–66, 69, 74, 76–77, 94–103

Quadriceps: 37–39, 52, 74–75

Iliotibial Bands: 37

Knee: 35–37, 49–53, 65–66, 75

Front of Lower Leg: 49, 75

Ankle: 34–37, 49–51, 65–66, 71–72, 91

Arch: 34, 50

Toes: 34, 50

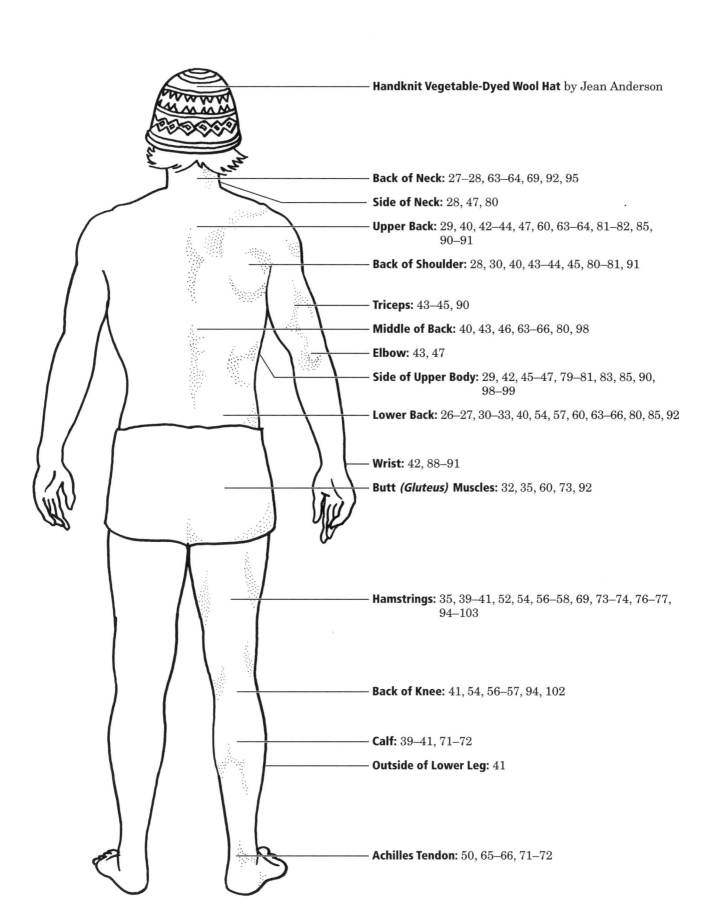

Handknit Vegetable-Dyed Wool Hat by Jean Anderson

Back of Neck: 27–28, 63–64, 69, 92, 95

Side of Neck: 28, 47, 80

Upper Back: 29, 40, 42–44, 47, 60, 63–64, 81–82, 85, 90–91

Back of Shoulder: 28, 30, 40, 43–44, 45, 80–81, 91

Triceps: 43–45, 90

Middle of Back: 40, 43, 46, 63–66, 80, 98

Elbow: 43, 47

Side of Upper Body: 29, 42, 45–47, 79–81, 83, 85, 90, 98–99

Lower Back: 26–27, 30–33, 40, 54, 57, 60, 63–66, 80, 85, 92

Wrist: 42, 88–91

Butt *(Gluteus)* **Muscles:** 32, 35, 60, 73, 92

Hamstrings: 35, 39–41, 52, 54, 56–58, 69, 73–74, 76–77, 94–103

Back of Knee: 41, 54, 56–57, 94, 102

Calf: 39–41, 71–72

Outside of Lower Leg: 41

Achilles Tendon: 50, 65–66, 71–72

Relaxing Stretches for Your Back

This is a series of very easy stretches that you can do lying on your back. This series is beneficial because each position stretches a body area that is generally hard to relax. You can use this routine for mild stretching and relaxation.

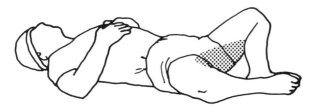

Relax, with knees bent and soles of your feet together. This comfortable position will stretch your groin. Hold for 30 seconds. Let the pull of gravity do the stretching. You may want to put a small pillow behind your head for comfort.

Variation: From this lying groin stretch, gently rock your legs as one unit (see dotted lines) back and forth about 10–12 times. These are real easy movements of no more than one inch in either direction. Initiate movements from top of your hips. This will gently limber up your groin and hips.

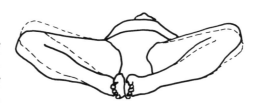

A Stretch for the Lower Back, Side, and Top of Hip

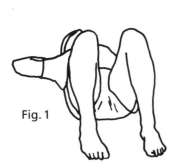

Fig. 1

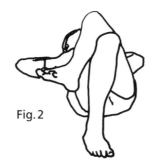

Fig. 2

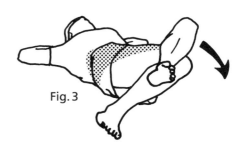

Fig. 3

Bring your knees together and rest your feet on the floor. Interlace your fingers behind your head with your arms on the floor (fig. 1). Now lift the left leg over the right leg (fig. 2). From here, use your left leg to pull your right leg toward the floor (fig. 3) until you feel a good stretch along the side of the hip or in the lower back. Relax. Keep the upper back, back of head, shoulders, and elbows flat on the floor. Hold for 10–20 seconds. *The idea is not to touch the floor with your right knee, but to stretch within **your** limits.* Repeat the stretch for the other side, crossing the right over the left leg and pulling down to the right. Exhale as you go into the stretch, then breath rhythmically as you stretch.

> • Do not hold your breath.
> • Breathe rhythmically.
> • Relax.

If you have sciatic* problems of the lower back, this stretch can help. But *be careful*. Hold only stretch tensions that feel good. Never stretch to the point of pain.

PNF Technique: *Contract—Relax—Stretch. (See pp. 206–209.)*

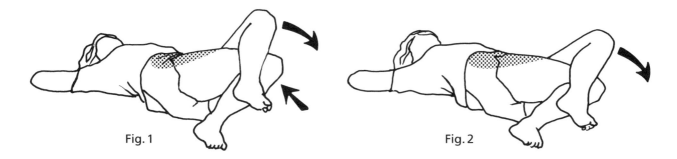

Fig. 1   Fig. 2

To do this, hold down the right leg with the left leg, as you try to pull the right leg back to an upright position. This contracts the muscles of the hip area *(fig. 1)*. Hold the contraction for 5 seconds, then relax and do the previous stretch *(fig. 2)*. This technique is good for people who are tight.

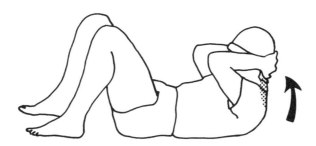

To reduce tension in the neck: While still lying on the floor, you can stretch your upper spine and neck. Interlace your fingers behind your head at about ear level. Slowly pull your head forward until you feel a slight stretch in the back of the neck. Hold for 3–5 seconds, then slowly return to the original starting position. Do this 3–4 times to loosen up the upper spine and neck gradually. Keep your jaw relaxed (back teeth slightly separated) and keep breathing.

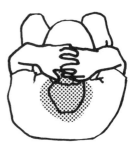

---

*The sciatic nerve is the longest and largest nerve of the body. It originates in the lumbar portion of the spine (lower back) and travels down the entire length of both legs and out to the great toe.

PNF Technique: *Contract — Relax — Stretch.* From a bent-knee position, interlace your fingers behind your head (not your neck). Before stretching the back of your neck, gently lift your head upward and forward off the floor. Then move the back of your head downward toward the floor as you resist this movement with your hands and arms. Hold this isometric contraction for 3–4 seconds. Relax for 1–2 seconds, then gently pull your head forward (as in the previous stretch), with your chin going toward your navel until you feel a mild, comfortable stretch. Hold for 3–5 seconds. Do 2–3 times.

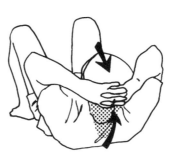

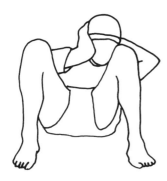

Gently pull your head and chin toward your left knee. Hold for 3–5 seconds. Relax and lower your head back down to the floor, then pull your head gently toward your right knee. Repeat 2–3 times.

With the back of your head on the floor, turn your chin toward your shoulder (as you keep your head resting on the floor). Turn your chin only as far as needed to get an easy stretch in the side of your neck. Hold for 3–5 seconds, then stretch to the other side. Repeat 2–3 times. Keep your jaw relaxed and don't hold your breath.

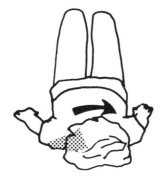

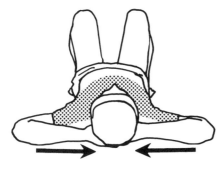

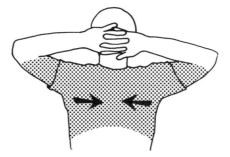

Shoulder Blade Pinch: Interlace your fingers behind your head and pull your shoulder blades together to create tension in the upper back area. (As you do this your chest should move upward.) Hold for 4–5 seconds, then relax and gently pull your head forward as shown on p. 27. This will also release tension in the neck.

Think of creating tension in the neck and shoulders, relaxing the same area, then stretching the back of the neck to help keep the muscles of the neck free to move without tightness. Repeat 3–4 times.

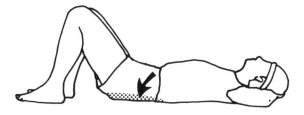

Lower Back Flattener: To relieve tension in your lower back, tighten your butt *(gluteus)* muscles and, at the same time, tighten your abdominal muscles to flatten your lower back. Hold this tension for 5–8 seconds, then relax. Repeat 2–3 times. Concentrate on maintaining constant muscle contraction. This pelvic tilting exercise will strengthen the butt *(gluteus)* and abdominal muscles so that you are able to sit and stand with good posture.

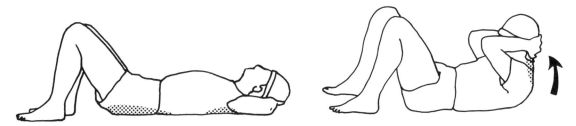

Shoulder Blade Pinch and Gluteus Tightener: Now, simultaneously do the shoulder blade pinch, flatten your lower back, and tighten your butt muscles. Hold contraction for 5 seconds, then relax and pull your head forward to stretch the back of your neck and upper back. Repeat 3–4 times. This feels great.

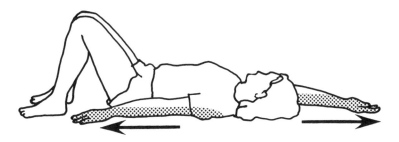

Now put one arm above your head (palm up) and the other arm down along your side (palm down). Reach in opposite directions at the same time to stretch your shoulders and back. Hold stretch for 6–8 seconds. Do both sides at least twice. Keep your lower back relaxed and flat. Keep your jaw relaxed.

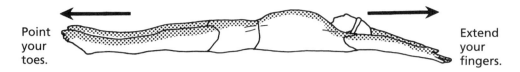

Point your toes.

Extend your fingers.

Elongation Stretches: Extend your arms overhead and straighten out your legs. Now reach as far as is comfortable in an opposite direction with your arms and legs. Stretch for 5 seconds, then relax.

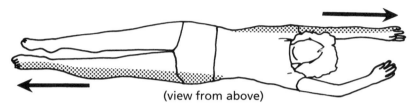

(view from above)

Now stretch diagonally. Point the toes of your left foot as you extend your right arm. Stretch as far as is comfortable. Hold for 5 seconds, then relax. Stretch the right leg and the left arm the same way. Hold each stretch for at least 5 seconds, then relax.

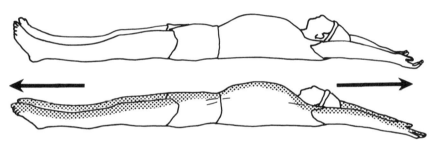

Now, at the same time, stretch both arms and both legs again. Hold for 5 seconds, then relax. This is a good stretch for the muscles of the rib cage, abdominals, spine, shoulders, arms, ankles, and feet.

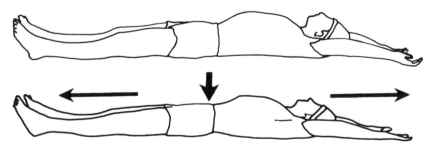

As a variation of this stretch, pull in with the abdominal muscles as you stretch. This will make you feel slim, and is a great exercise for your internal organs.

Doing these elongation stretches three times will reduce tension and tightness and relax your spine and entire body. They help reduce overall body tension quickly. You could do these just before sleeping.

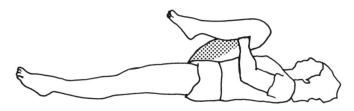

Pull your right leg toward your chest with hands behind the knee. For this stretch keep the back of your head on the floor or mat if possible, but don't strain. Hold an easy stretch for 10–30 seconds. Repeat, pulling your left leg toward your chest. Be sure to keep your lower back flat. If no real stretch is felt, don't worry. If the position feels good, use it. This is a very good position for the legs, feet, and back.

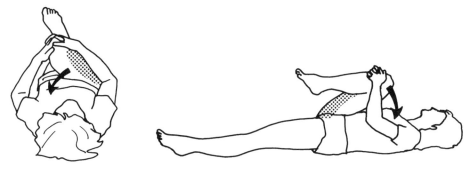

Variation: Pull your knee to your chest, then pull the knee and leg across your body toward your opposite shoulder to create a stretch on the outside of your right hip. Hold an easy stretch for 10–20 seconds. Do both sides.

Variation: From a lying position, gently pull your right knee toward the outside of the right shoulder. Your hands should be placed on the back of your leg, just above your knee. Hold for 10–20 seconds. Breathe continuously and deeply. Repeat for the other leg.

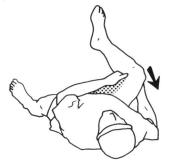

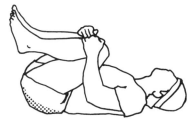 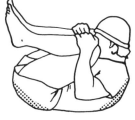

After pulling one leg at a time to your chest, pull both legs to your chest. This time concentrate on keeping the back of your head down and then curling your head up toward your knees.

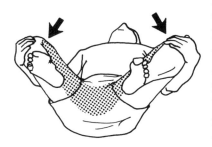

Lie on your back with your knees flexed toward your chest. Place your hands on your lower legs just below your knees. To stretch the insides of your upper legs and groin area, slowly pull your legs out and down until you feel a mild stretch. Hold for 10 seconds. The back of your head can be flat on the floor, resting on a small pillow or up off the floor so that you can look between your legs.

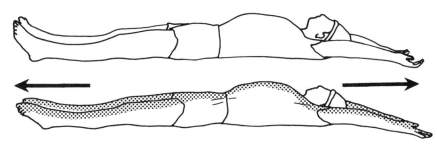

Straighten out both legs again. Stretch and then relax.

A Stretch for the Lower Back and Side of Hip

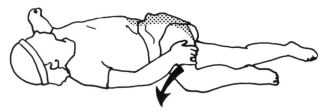

Bend your left knee at 90° and, with your right hand, pull that bent leg up and over your other leg as shown above. Turn your head to look toward the hand of the left arm that is straight out from the shoulder (head should be resting on floor, not held up). Now, using the right hand on your left thigh (resting just above knee) pull your bent (left) leg down toward the floor until you get a mild stretch feeling in your lower back and side of hip. Relax your feet and ankles and keep the back of your shoulders flat on the floor. Hold an easy stretch for 15–20 seconds, each side.

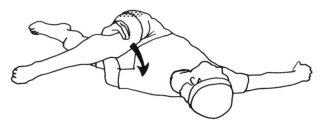

To increase the stretch in your buttocks, reach under your right leg and behind your knee. Slowly pull your right knee toward your opposite shoulder until you get a mild stretch. Keep both shoulders flat on the floor. Hold for 15–20 seconds. Do both legs.

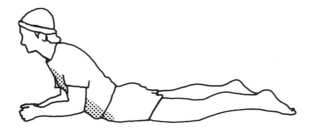

Back Extension: Starting from a prone position (lying on your stomach), place your elbows beneath your shoulders. A mild tension should be felt in the middle to lower back area. Keep the front of the hips on the floor. Hold for 5–10 seconds. Repeat 2–3 times.

You can end a series of stretches for your back by lying in the "fetus position." Lie on your side with your legs curled up and your head resting on your hands. Relax.

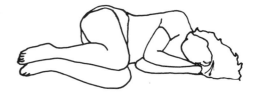

SUMMARY OF STRETCHES FOR YOUR BACK

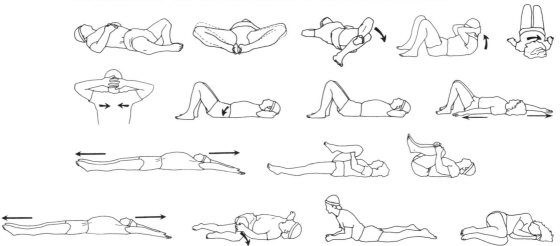

Do these stretches, in this order, to relax your back.

Learn to listen to your body. If the stretch builds or you feel pain, your body is trying to let you know that something is wrong, that there is a problem. If this happens, ease off gradually until the stretch feels right.

Stretches for the Legs, Feet, and Ankles

Rotate your ankle clockwise and counterclockwise through a complete range of motion with slight resistance provided by your hand. This rotary motion helps to gently stretch out tight ankle ligaments. Repeat 10–20 times in each direction. Do with both ankles and feel if there is any difference between ankles in terms of tightness and range of motion. Sometimes an ankle that has been sprained will feel a bit weaker and tighter. This difference may go unnoticed until you work each ankle separately and make a comparison.

Next, use your fingers to gently pull the toes toward you to stretch the top of the foot and tendons of the toes. Hold an easy stretch for 10 seconds. Repeat 2–3 times. Do both feet. Holding this position also helps relax the bottom of the foot *(plantar fascia)*.

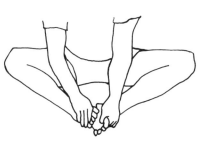

Place your thumbs at the base of your large toes (bottom of feet where toes come out of the foot), index fingers slightly bent, and placed over the nails of your large toes. Use your fingers and thumbs to move your large toes back and forth for 15–20 seconds, then rotate your large toes in a circular motion both clockwise and counterclockwise for 10–15 seconds. Concentrate on increasing the range of motion of your toes as you manipulate this area. A great way to improve or maintain the flexibility and circulation of this area.

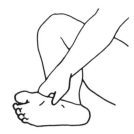

With your thumbs, massage up and down the longitudinal arch of your foot. Use circular motions with a good amount of pressure to loosen tissues. Do both feet. This should help reduce the tension and tightness in the feet.

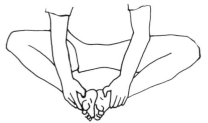

Variation: Massage the arches of your feet with your thumbs. Move up and down the arches, working out sore areas with circular massage. This is good to do while watching TV or just before going to sleep. Massage with pressure that feels good.

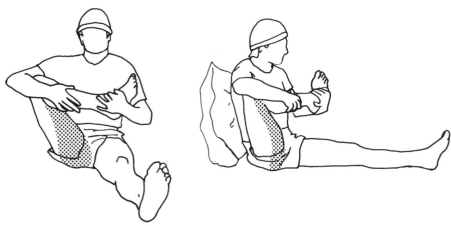

To stretch the upper hamstrings and hip, hold onto the outside of your ankle with one hand, with your other hand and forearm around your bent knee. Gently pull the leg *as one unit* toward your chest until you feel an easy stretch in the back of the upper leg. You may want to rest your back against something for support. Hold for 10–20 seconds. Make sure the leg is pulled as one unit so that stress is not felt in the knee. Slightly increase the stretch by pulling the leg a little closer to your chest. Hold this developmental stretch for 10 seconds. Do both sides. Is one leg more flexible than the other?

For some of you, this position will not provide a stretch. If that is the case, do the stretch shown below.

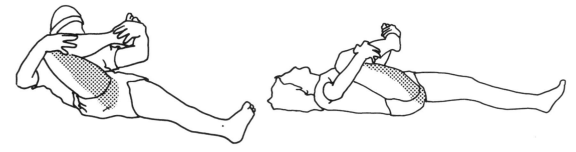

Begin by lying down, then lean forward to hold onto your leg as described in the previous stretch. Gently pull your leg as one unit toward your chest until you feel an easy stretch in the butt and upper hamstring. Hold for 20 seconds. Doing this stretch in a lying position will increase the stretch in the hamstrings for people who are relatively flexible in this area. Do both legs and compare.

Experiment: See the difference in the stretch when your head is forward and when the back of your head is on the floor. Always keep every stretch within a personal comfort range. You can place a small pillow behind your head for comfort.

Lie on your back. Bend your right knee and put the outside of your right lower leg just above your opposite knee. With your hands just below your left knee, gently pull your leg toward your chest until a stretch is felt in your buttocks area *(piriformis)*. Hold for 15–20 seconds. Stretch both legs. Lift the back of your head off the floor and look straight ahead as you stretch. Breathe slowly and deeply.

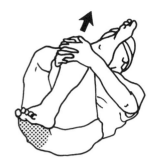

PNF Technique: *Contract—Relax—Stretch.* Another way to stretch the buttocks is to use the contract-relax-stretch technique. Starting from the previous position, move your left leg downward as you resist movement (contraction) for 4–5 seconds. Then relax and stretch for 15–20 seconds as previously described. A really good stretch for the *piriformis.*

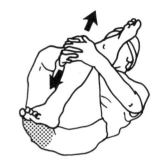

Lie on your left side and rest the side of your head in the palm of your left hand. Hold the top of your right foot with your right hand between the toes and ankle joint. Gently pull the right heel toward the right buttock to stretch the ankle and quadriceps (front of thigh). Hold an easy stretch for 10 seconds.

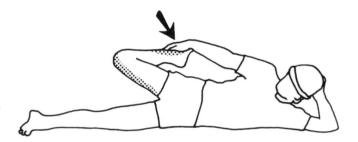

Never stretch the knee to the point of pain. Always be in control.

Now move the front of your right hip forward by contracting the right thigh *(quadriceps)* muscles as you push your right foot into your right hand. This should stretch the front of your thigh and relax your hamstrings. Hold an easy stretch for 10 seconds. Keep the body in a straight line. Now stretch the left leg in the same way. (You may also get a good stretch in the front of the shoulder.) At first it may be hard to hold this for very long. Just work on the proper way to stretch without worrying about flexibility or how you look. Stretching regularly will create a positive change. I like to follow this stretch with the hamstrings stretch at the top of page 58.

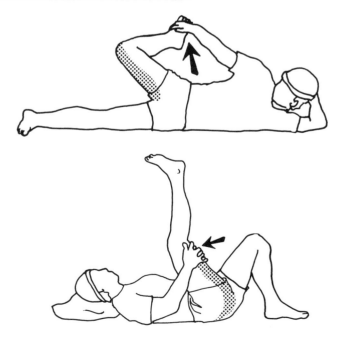

Stretching Your Iliotibial Bands

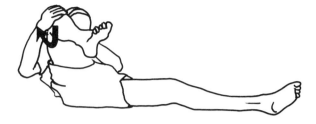

Lie on your side while holding the front of your lower leg from the outside with your right hand. Circle your leg in front of you, then slightly behind you. As you circle your leg, move your right hand to the top of your right ankle.

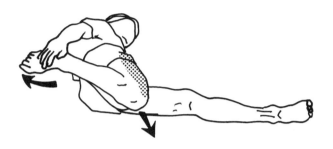

Now you should be on your side as in the figure to the left. To stretch the iliotibial band, gently pull your right heel toward your buttocks as you move the inside of your knee downward toward the floor. You should feel a stretch on the outside of your upper leg. Hold for 15–20 seconds. Do both legs.

If you experience any knee pain with these stretches, don't do them. Instead, use the opposite-hand-to-opposite-foot technique of stretching the knee (p. 75).

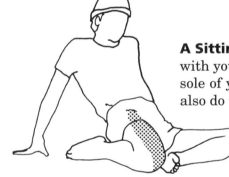

A Sitting Stretch for the Quadriceps: First sit with your right leg bent, with your right heel just outside your right hip. The left leg is bent and the sole of your left foot is next to the inside of your upper right leg. (You can also do this stretch with your left leg straight out in front of you.)

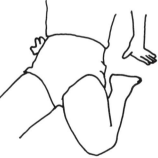

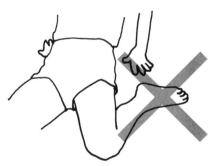

Your foot should be extended back with the ankle flexed. If your ankle is too tight, move your foot just enough to the side to lessen the tension in your ankle.

Do not let your foot flare out to the side in this position. By keeping your foot pointed straight back, you take the stress off the inside of your knee. The more your foot flares to the side, the more stress there is on your knee.

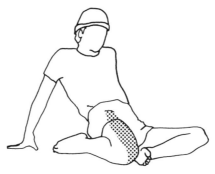

Now, slowly lean *straight back* until you feel an easy stretch. Use your hands for balance and support. Hold this easy stretch for 10–15 seconds.

Some people will have to lean back a lot further than others to find the right stretch tension. And some people may feel the right stretch without leaning back at all. Be aware of how you feel and forget about how far you can go. Stretch to where you are comfortable and don't worry about anyone else.

Do not let your knee lift off the floor or mat. If your knee comes up, you are leaning back too far and overstretching. Ease up on the stretch.

> Be sure to hold only stretches that are comfortable.
> **Be careful to not overstretch.**

Now slowly, and in complete control and comfort, increase into the developmental stretch. Hold for 10 seconds, then slowly come out of it. Switch sides and stretch the left thigh the same way.

Can you feel any difference in tension? Is one side more limber than the other? Are you more flexible on one side?

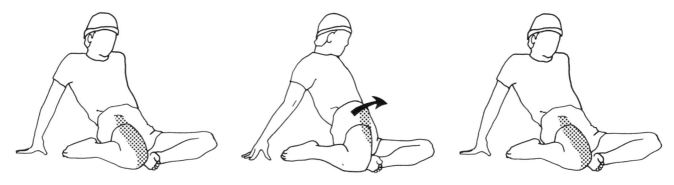

After stretching your quads, practice tightening the buttocks on the side of the bent leg as you turn the hip over. This will help stretch the front of your hip *(iliopsoas)* and give a better overall stretch to upper thigh area. After contracting the butt *(gluteus)* muscles for 5–8 seconds, let the buttocks relax. Drop your hip down and continue to stretch the quads for another 10–15 seconds. Practice to eventually get both sides of the buttocks to touch the floor at the same time during this stretch. Now do the other side.

Note: Stretching the quads first, then turning the hip over as the buttocks contract will help change the stretch feeling when you return to the original quads stretch.

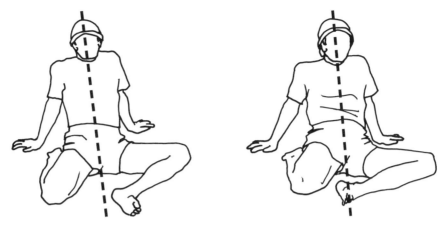

If this produces pain in the knee, move the knee of the leg being stretched closer to the midline of your body until it's more comfortable. Moving this way may take the stress off the knee, but if there is continuing pain, stop doing this stretch.

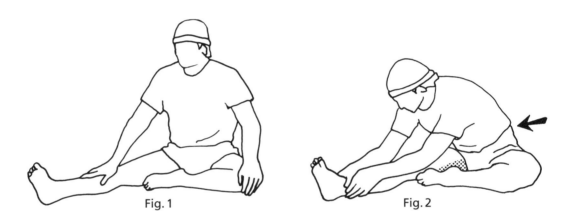

Fig. 1   Fig. 2

To stretch the hamstrings of the same leg that was bent (see previous page), straighten the right leg with the sole of your left foot slightly touching the inside of your right thigh. You are now in the straight-leg, bent-knee position *(fig. 1)*. Slowly bend forward from the hips toward the foot of the straight leg *(fig. 2)* until you create the slightest feeling of stretch tension. Hold for 10–15 seconds. After the stretch tension has diminished, bend forward from the hips a bit more. Exhale as you hold this developmental stretch for 10 seconds, breathing rhythmically. Then switch sides and stretch the left leg in the same manner.

During this stretch, keep the foot of the straight leg upright, with the ankle and toes relaxed. Be sure the quadriceps are soft to the touch (relaxed). Do not dip your head forward when initiating the stretch.

I have found that it is best to stretch your quads first, then the hamstrings of the same leg. It is easier to stretch the hamstrings after the quadriceps have been stretched.

Use a towel or elastic cord to help you stretch if you cannot *easily* reach your foot.

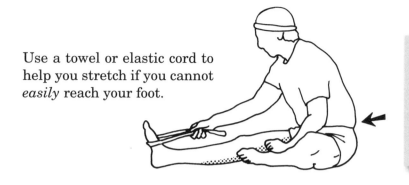

Get used to doing variations of basic stretches. In each variation you will use your body in a different way. You will become more aware of all the stretch possibilities when you change the angles of the stretch tension, even if the angle changes are very slight.

Variations of the Straight-leg, Bent-knee Position

Reach across your body with your left arm to the outside of your right leg. Place your right hand out to the side for balance. This will stretch the muscles of the upper back and spine and the side of the lower back, as well as the hamstrings. To change the stretch, look over your right shoulder as you turn the front of your left hip slightly to the inside. This will stretch the lower back and in between the shoulder blades. Breathe easily. Do not hold your breath. Hold for 10–15 seconds.

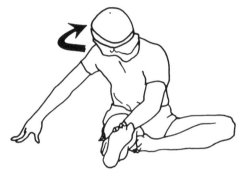

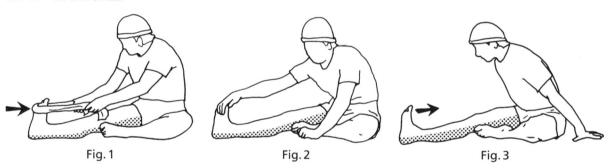

| Fig. 1 | Fig. 2 | Fig. 3 |

To stretch the back of the lower leg (calf and *soleus* muscles), use a towel around the ball of your foot to pull your toes toward your knee (*fig. 1*) or if you are more flexible, use your hand to pull your toes toward your knee (*fig. 2*). Or pull your foot toward your knee (dorsiflexion) without using your hand, and hold, then lean slightly forward to stretch your calf (*fig. 3*). Hold for 10–20 seconds.

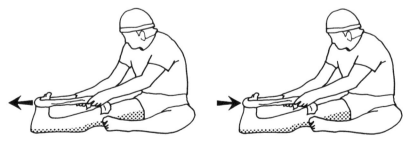

PNF Technique: *Contract—Relax—Stretch.* Another way to stretch the back of your lower leg is to first contract this area by pushing your foot downward as you resist with a towel for 4 to 5 seconds. Then relax. Now use the towel to pull your foot toward your knee. Hold for 10–15 seconds.

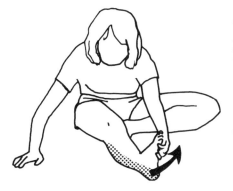

To stretch the outside of your lower leg, reach down with your opposite hand and hold onto the outside border of your foot (see drawing). Now, gently turn the outside of your foot to the inside to feel a stretch on the outside of your lower leg. This stretch can be done with a straight leg, or it can be done with your leg flexed at your knee if you are unable to *easily* hold onto the outside border of your foot with your leg straight. In the straight-leg position the quadriceps should be soft and relaxed. Hold an easy stretch for 10 seconds.

> Never lock your knees when doing sitting stretches. Be sure to keep the front of your thigh *(quadriceps)* relaxed in all positions using a straight leg. You can't stretch the hamstrings correctly when the opposing set of muscles (the quadriceps) are not relaxed.

SUMMARY OF STRETCHES FOR THE LEGS, FEET, AND ANKLES

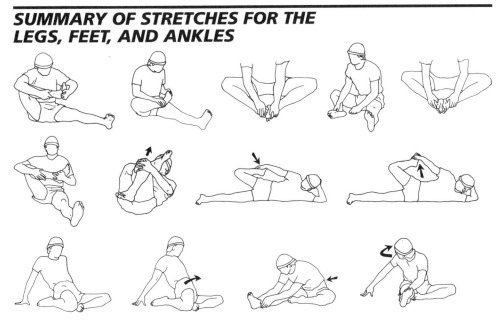

Do these stretches, in this order, as a routine.

> Bouncing while stretching can actually make you tighter, rather than more flexible. For example, if you bounce four or five times while touching your toes, then bend over again several minutes later, you'll probably find that you are farther away from your toes than when you started! Each bouncing movement activates the stretch reflex, tightening the very muscles you are trying to stretch.

Stretches for the Back, Shoulders, and Arms

There are many stretches that can reduce tension and increase flexibility in the upper body. Most of the sitting or standing stretches can be done anywhere.

Many people suffer from tension in the upper body because of stress in their lives. Quite a few muscular athletes are stiff in the upper body because of not stretching that area.

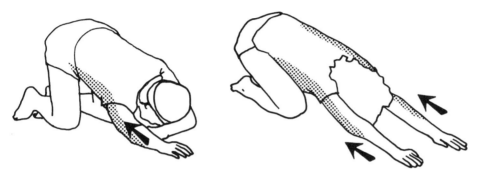

With legs bent under you, reach forward with your hands, then pull back with straight arms while you press down slightly with your palms.

You can do this stretch one arm at a time or both at the same time. Pulling with just one arm provides more control and isolates the stretch on either side. You should feel this in your shoulders, arms, lats (*latissimus dorsi*) or sides, upper back, and even your lower back. When you do this for the first time, you may feel it only in the shoulders and arms, but as you do it more you will learn to stretch other areas; by slightly moving your hips in either direction, you can increase or decrease the stretch. Don't strain. Be relaxed. Hold for 15 seconds.

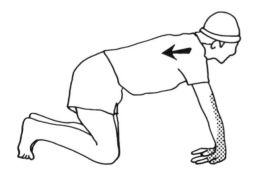

A Forearm and Wrist Stretch: Support yourself on your hands and knees. Thumbs should be pointed to the outside, with fingers pointed toward knees. Keep palms flat as you lean back to stretch the front part of your forearms. Hold an easy stretch for 10–20 seconds. Relax, then stretch again. You may find you are very tight in this area.

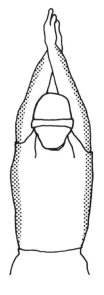

Keep your knees slightly flexed during standing upper-body stretches.

With arms extended overhead and palms together as drawing shows, stretch your arms upward and slightly backward. Breathe in as you stretch upward. Hold for 5–8 seconds, as you breathe easily.

This is a great stretch for the muscles of the outer portions of the arms, shoulders, and ribs. It can be done any time and any place to relieve tension and create a feeling of relaxation and well-being.

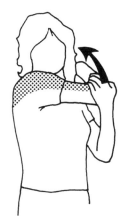

Remember: Keep your jaw relaxed and breathe deeply as you stretch.

To stretch your shoulder and the middle of your upper back, gently pull your elbow across your chest toward your opposite shoulder. Hold for 10 seconds.

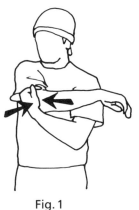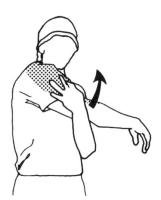

Fig. 1   Fig. 2

PNF Technique: *Contract—Relax—Stretch.* Stand with knees slightly flexed. With your left hand, hold the outside of your right arm just above your elbow. Move your right arm away from your body as you resist with your left hand. Hold an isometric contraction for 3–4 seconds *(fig. 1).* After relaxing a moment, gently pull your right arm across your body toward your shoulder until you feel a comfortable stretch in the outside of your shoulder and upper arm *(fig. 2).* Hold for 10 seconds, then repeat to other side.

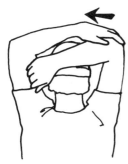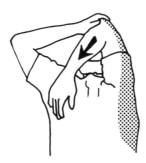

Here is a simple stretch for your triceps and the top of your shoulders. With arms overhead, hold the elbow of one arm with the hand of the other arm. Gently pull the elbow behind your head, creating a stretch. Do it slowly. Hold for 15 seconds. Do not hold your breath.

Stretch both sides. Does it feel as if one side is a lot tighter than the other side? This is a good way to begin loosening up your arms and shoulders. You can do this stretch while walking.

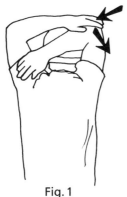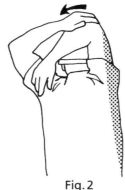

Fig. 1   Fig. 2

PNF Technique: *Contract—Relax—Stretch.* Stand with your knees slightly flexed and your feet about shoulder-width apart. Hold your right elbow with your left hand. Move your right elbow downward as you resist this movement with your left hand (isometric contraction) for 3–4 seconds *(fig. 1)*. After relaxing a moment, gently pull your elbow over, behind your head until you feel a mild stretch in the back of your upper arm as in the previous stretch *(fig. 2)*. Hold for 10–15 seconds. Repeat to other side.

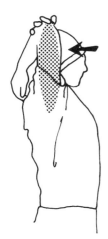

Start in a standing position with your knees slightly flexed. Bend your right elbow and put your arm behind your head. Hold onto your right elbow with your left hand. To stretch the armpit area and shoulder move the back of your head back against your right arm, until a mild stretch is felt. Hold for 10–15 seconds. Do both sides.

Variation: From a standing position, with your knees slightly bent (1 inch), gently pull your elbow behind your head as you bend from your hips to the side. Hold an easy stretch for 10 seconds. Do both sides. *Keep your knees slightly bent for better balance.* Do not hold your breath.

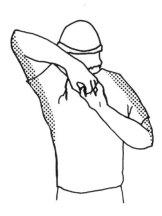

Another Shoulder Stretch: Reach behind your head and down as far as you can with your left hand and, if you are able, grab your right hand coming up, palm out. Grab your fingers and hold for 5–10 seconds. If your hands do not meet, try one of the following:

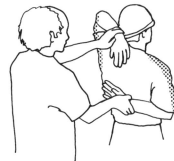

Have someone pull your hands slowly toward each other until you get an easy stretch and hold it. Do not stretch too far. You may get a great stretch without touching your fingers. Stretch within *your* limits.

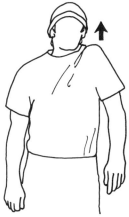

Or drop a towel behind your head. With your upper arm bent, reach up with your other arm to hold onto the end of the towel. Gradually move your hand up on the towel, pulling your upper arm downwards.

Work a little on it every day and get a good stretch. After a while you will be able to do this stretch without help. It reduces tension and increases flexibility. It also acts as an upper body revitalizer when you are tired.

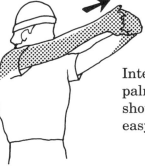

Interlace your fingers out in front of you at shoulder height. Turn your palms outward as you extend your arms forward to feel a stretch in your shoulders, middle of upper back, arms, hands, fingers, and wrists. Hold an easy stretch for 15 seconds, then relax and repeat.

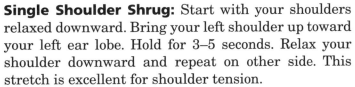

Single Shoulder Shrug: Start with your shoulders relaxed downward. Bring your left shoulder up toward your left ear lobe. Hold for 3–5 seconds. Relax your shoulder downward and repeat on other side. This stretch is excellent for shoulder tension.

PNF Technique: Contract—Relax—Stretch.

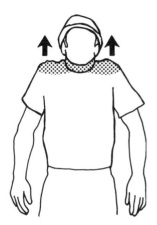

Shoulder Shrug: First, raise the top of your shoulders toward your ears until you feel a slight tension in your neck and shoulders. Hold for 5 seconds. Then relax shoulders downward. Think: "Shoulders hang, shoulders down."

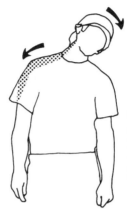

Then gently lower your right shoulder downward as you lean your head, with your ear toward your left shoulder. Hold a comfortable stretch for 5 seconds, then repeat on your other side.

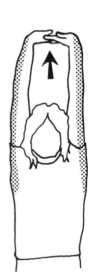

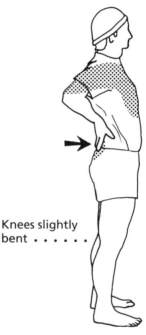

Knees slightly bent . . . . . .

Now interlace your fingers above your head and, with your palms facing upward, push your arms slightly back and up. Feel the stretch in your arms, shoulders, and upper back. Hold for 15 seconds. Do not hold your breath. This stretch is good to do anywhere, anytime, and is excellent for slumping shoulders. Breathe deeply.

Standing with your knees slightly bent, place your palms on your lower back just above your hips, fingers pointing downward. Gently push your palms forward to create an extension in the lower back. Hold for 10 seconds. Repeat twice. Use this stretch after sitting for an extended period of time. Do not hold your breath.

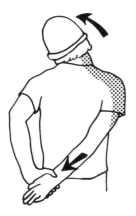

To stretch the side of your neck, lean your head sideways toward your left shoulder as your left hand pulls your right arm down and across, behind your back. Hold an easy stretch for 10–15 seconds. Do both sides.

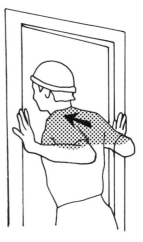

Stand in a doorway and place your hands at about shoulder-height on either side of the doorway. Move your upper body forward until you feel a comfortable stretch in your arms and chest. Keep your chest and head up and knees slightly bent while doing this stretch. Hold for 15 seconds.

The next stretches are done with your fingers interlaced behind your back.

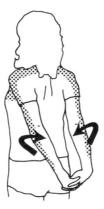

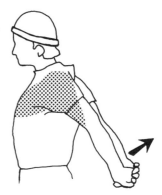

For the first stretch, slowly turn your elbows inward while straightening your arms. This stretches the shoulders, arms, and chest. Hold for 5–10 seconds.

If that is fairly easy, then lift your arms up behind you until you feel a stretch in the arms, shoulders, or chest. Hold an easy stretch for 5–10 seconds. This is good to do when you find yourself slumping forward from the shoulders. Keep your chest out and chin in. This stretch can be done any time.

SUMMARY OF STRETCHES FOR BACK, SHOULDERS, AND ARMS

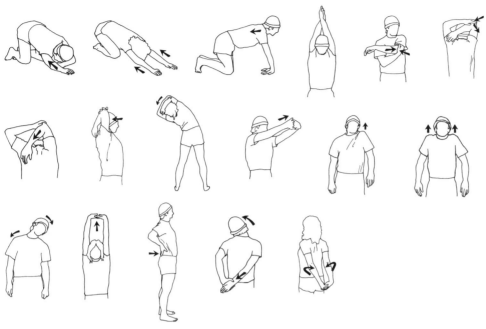

You can do these stretches, in this order, as a routine.

It is better to understretch than to overstretch. Always be at a point where you can stretch further, and never at a point where you have gone as far as you can go.

A Series of Stretches for the Legs

Toe Pointer: This is another good stretch for the legs. You can do a series of stretches for the legs, feet, and groin from the toe pointer position.

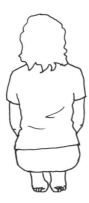

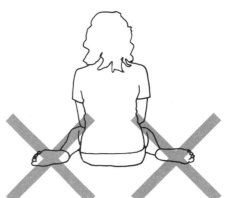

This position helps stretch the knees, ankles, and quadriceps. The toe pointer will also help relax the calves so they may be stretched more easily.

Do not let your feet flare out to the sides when doing this stretch. A flared-out position of the lower legs and feet may cause overstretching of the inside (medial collateral) ligaments of the knee.

Caution: If you have or have had knee problems, be very careful bending the knees underneath you. Do it slowly and under control. If there is any pain, discontinue the stretch.

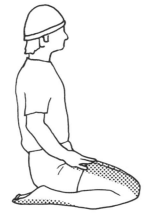

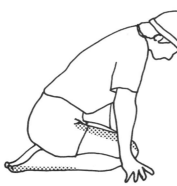

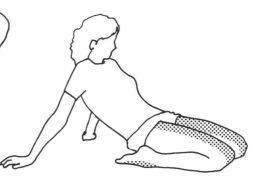

Most women will not feel much of a stretch in this position. But for tight people, especially men, this position lets you know if you have tight ankles. If there is a strain, place your hands on the outside of your legs for support as you balance yourself slightly forward. Find a position you can hold for 20–30 seconds.

If you are tight, do not overstretch. Regularity in stretching creates positive change. There will be noticeable improvement in ankle flexibility within several weeks.

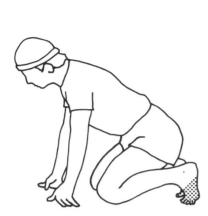
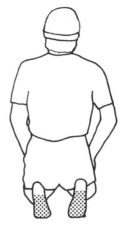

Variation: To stretch your toes and the bottom of your foot *(plantar fascia)*, sit with your toes underneath you *(see above)*. Put your hands in front of you for balance and control. If you want to stretch further, slowly lean backwards until it feels right. Hold only stretches that feel good and you can control. Stretch easily for 5–10 seconds. Be careful. There may be a lot of tension in this part of the foot and toes. Be patient. Gradually get your body used to changing by stretching regularly. Return to toe pointer after doing this stretch.

To Stretch the Achilles Tendon Area and Ankles

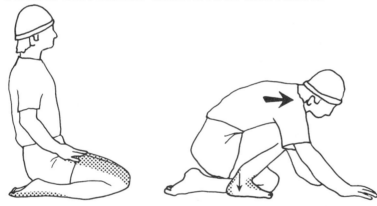

Bring the toes of one foot almost even with or parallel to the knee of the other leg. Let the heel of the bent leg come off the ground one-half inch or so. Lower your heel toward the ground while leaning forward on your thigh (just above the knee) with your chest and shoulder. The idea is not to get the heel flat, but to use the forward pressure from your shoulder on your thigh to gently stretch the Achilles tendon area. Be careful. The Achilles tendon area needs only a *very slight stretch*. Hold for 5–10 seconds.

This stretch is great for tight ankles and arches. Be sure to work both sides. Here again, you will probably find that one side is more flexible than the other.

> As we get older or go through periods of inactivity and then are active again, there is a lot of stress and strain on the lower legs, ankles, and arches. One way to reduce or eliminate the pain and soreness of new activity is to stretch before and after exercise.

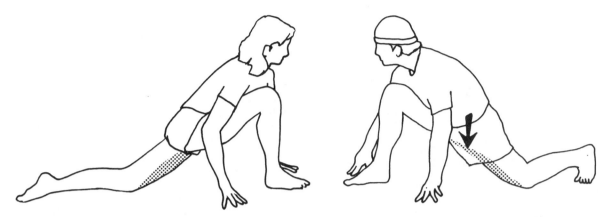

To stretch the muscles in the front of the hip *(iliopsoas)*, move one leg forward until the knee of the forward leg is directly over the ankle. Your other knee should be resting on the floor. Now, without changing the position of the knee on the floor or the forward foot, lower the front of your hip downward to create an easy stretch. Hold for 15–20 seconds. You should feel this stretch in the front of the hip and possibly in the hamstrings and groin.

Do not have your knee forward of the ankle. This will hinder the proper stretching of the hip and legs. The greater distance there is between the back knee and the heel of the front foot, the easier it is to stretch the hips and legs.

Variations: Turn the left hip slowly to the inside to change the area of the stretch. By only slightly changing angles, you are able to stretch many different, adjacent areas of the body. Hold an easy stretch for 10–20 seconds. Stretch both legs. This is excellent for the hips, lower back, and groin. You can look over your shoulder, behind you, to stretch your neck and upper back.

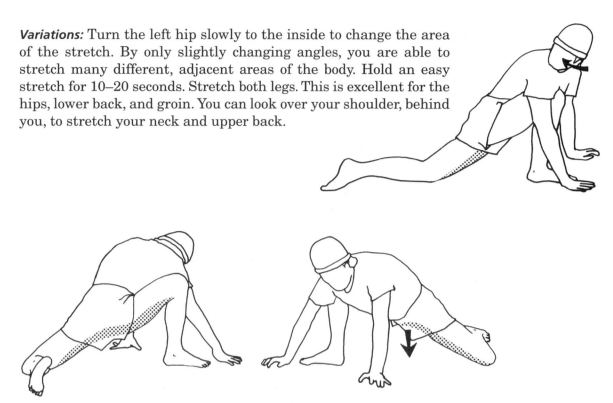

From the previous hip stretch you can isolate a stretch for the inside of the upper leg. Bend your rear knee and move your rear foot to the inside. This will make a 90° angle at the knee joint. Now move your shoulders off your knee and put your hands to the inside of your body for support. Move your hips downward to stretch the inside of your upper leg (groin). Do not move your back knee or front foot. Be sure that your front knee is directly above your ankle. Hold an easy stretch for 10–15 seconds. Try on the other side. Stretch both legs.

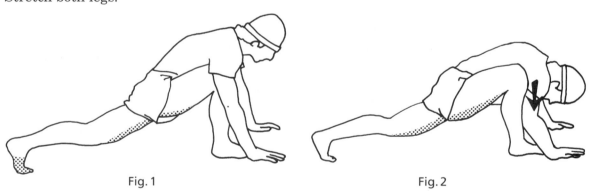

Fig. 1   Fig. 2

An excellent stretch for hip flexibility: With your front knee directly above your ankle, shift your weight up onto the toes and ball of your back foot *(fig. 1)*. Now hold an easy stretch with a fairly straight back leg for 15–20 seconds. Think of the front of your hip going down to create the right stretch tension. Use your hands for balance. This stretches the groin, hamstrings, and hip, and possibly behind the knee of the back leg. Do both legs.

Another variation is to change the stretch by gently lowering your upper body to the inside of the knee of the forward leg *(fig. 2)*. Hold a comfortable stretch for 15–20 seconds.

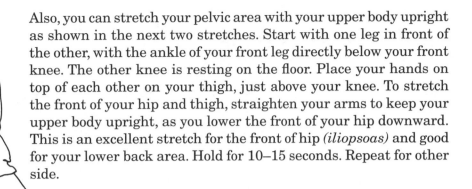

Also, you can stretch your pelvic area with your upper body upright as shown in the next two stretches. Start with one leg in front of the other, with the ankle of your front leg directly below your front knee. The other knee is resting on the floor. Place your hands on top of each other on your thigh, just above your knee. To stretch the front of your hip and thigh, straighten your arms to keep your upper body upright, as you lower the front of your hip downward. This is an excellent stretch for the front of hip *(iliopsoas)* and good for your lower back area. Hold for 10–15 seconds. Repeat for other side.

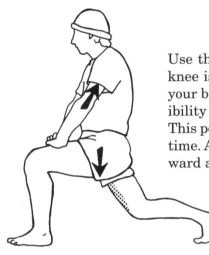

Use the same technique as in the last stretch, except your back knee is off the floor and you are on the ball of your foot, making your back leg much straighter. This stretch further promotes flexibility in the pelvis/hip area. Hold for 10–15 seconds. Do both sides. This position will challenge you to balance and stretch at the same time. As in the previous stretch, lower the front of your hip downward as you keep your torso upright (vertical).

SUMMARY OF STRETCHES FOR LEGS

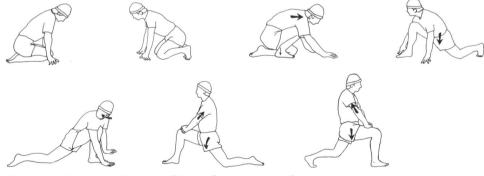

Do these leg stretches, in this order, as a routine.

Stretches for the Lower Back, Hips, Groin, and Hamstrings

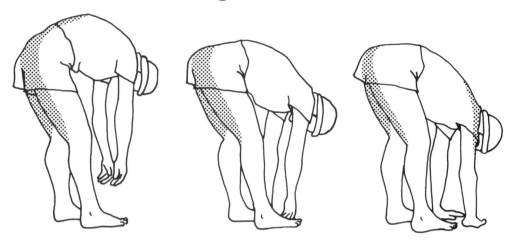

Start in a standing position with your feet about shoulder-width apart and pointed straight ahead. Slowly bend forward from the hips. *Keep your knees slightly bent* (1 inch) during the stretch so your lower back is not stressed. Let your neck and arms relax. Go to the point where you feel a slight stretch in the back of your legs. Stretch in this easy phase for 10–15 seconds, until you are relaxed. Let yourself relax physically by mentally concentrating on the area being stretched. Do not stretch with your knees locked, or bounce when you stretch. Simply hold an easy stretch.

> Stretch by how you *feel* and not by how *far* you can go.

When you do this stretch, you will feel it mostly in your hamstrings (back of thighs) and back of the knees. Your back will also be stretched, but you will feel this stretch mostly in the back of your legs.

Coming Back to an Upright Position

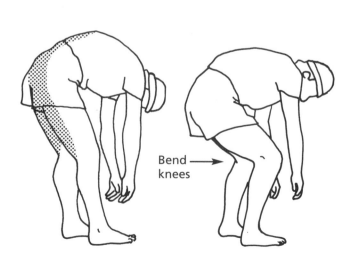

Bend → knees

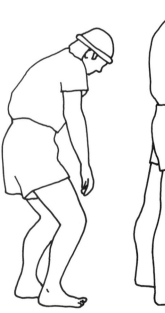

Important: Whenever you bend at the waist to stretch, remember to bend your knees slightly (1 inch or so). It takes the pressure off your lower back. Use the big muscles of the upper legs to stand up, instead of the small muscles of the lower back. Never bring yourself to an upright position with knees locked.

This principle is also important in lifting heavy objects off the ground (*see pp. 202–205,* Caring for Your Back).

> Stretching is not competitive. You may well not be able to touch your toes. The point is for *you* to get more flexible, not to stretch as far as others.

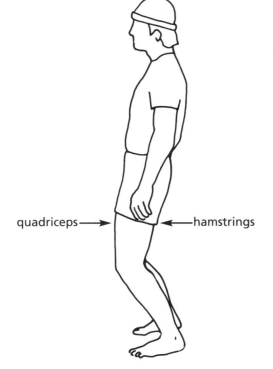

quadriceps→ ←hamstrings

PNF Technique: *Contract—Relax—Stretch.* Next, assume a bent-knee position with your heels flat, toes pointed straight ahead, and feet about shoulder-width apart. Hold for 30 seconds. In this bent-knee position, you are contracting the quadriceps and relaxing the hamstrings. The primary function of the quadriceps is to straighten the leg. The basic function of the hamstrings is to bend the knee. Because these muscles have opposing actions, contracting the quadriceps will relax the hamstrings.

As you hold this bent-knee position, feel the difference between the front and the back of your thigh. The quadriceps should feel hard and tight, while the hamstrings should feel soft and relaxed. It's easier to stretch the hamstrings if they are first relaxed.

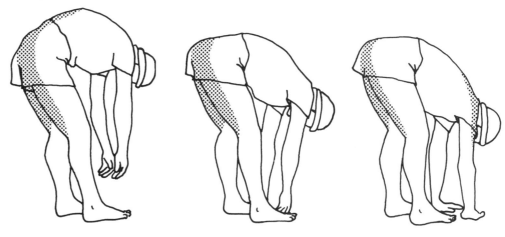

After holding the bent-knee position, stand up and then bend down again with knees slightly bent (1 inch). Don't bounce. You probably can go a little farther already. Hold about 10–15 seconds.

You must be in a comfortable and stable position when you stretch.

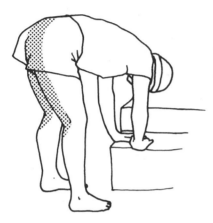

You will find it easier to hold this stretch if you can distribute your weight between your arms and legs. If you are unable to reach your toes (or ankles) with your knees slightly bent (many people cannot), then use a stair or curb, or a pile of books to rest your hands on. Find a balance between your hands and feet so you can relax.

Variation: With your hands, hold onto the back of your lower legs in the calf or ankle area. By pulling your upper body downward (gently!) with your hands, you will be able to increase the stretch in your legs and back, while you concentrate on relaxing in a very stable position. Do not go too far. Relax and stretch. Keep your knees slightly bent.

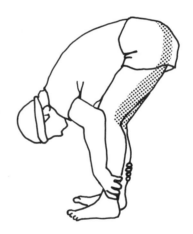

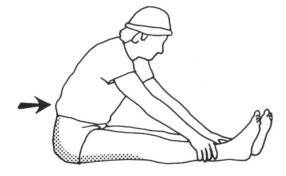

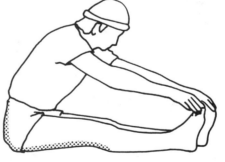

Next, sit down with your legs straight and feet upright, heels no more than six inches apart. Bend from the hips to get an easy stretch. Hold for 10–15 seconds. You will probably feel this just behind your knees and in the back of your upper legs. You may also feel a stretch in the lower back if your back is tight.

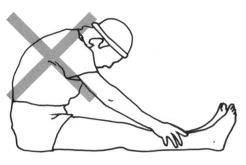

Do not dip your head forward as you begin this stretch. Try to keep your hips from rolling backwards.

Think of bending from your hips without rounding your upper back.

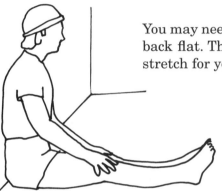

You may need to sit against a wall to keep your lower back flat. This position in itself may be enough of a stretch for you if you are extremely tight.

If you have trouble relaxing while doing this stretch, use a towel to help. Pull yourself forward (gently!) from the hips to where you can relax and still get a stretch. Use your hands and arms to pull yourself forward. Work your way down the towel with your fingers, until the stretch feels right. Be careful here. Do not overstretch.

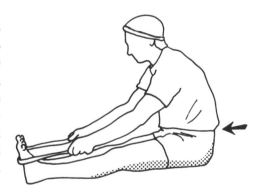

If this stretch seems to put pressure on your lower back, or you have had lower back problems, do the stretches shown on pages 39 and 58. These will feel more comfortable.

Be careful when you stretch with both legs in front of you or when bending forward at the hips in a standing position. You must not overstretch in these positions. Since the back of each leg probably differs in tightness and tension, don't stretch both legs at the same time if you have lower back problems. When one or both legs are extremely tight, it's difficult to stretch both legs at the same time and get the correct stretch for each leg. It is easier on your back to stretch each leg separately.

Lie on your back and lift your leg up toward a 90° angle at the thigh joint. Keep the lower back flat against the floor. Hold for 15–20 seconds. Repeat for other leg. If necessary, hold onto the back of your leg to create the stretch. Or put a towel or elastic cord around the bottom of your foot and pull gently. Only stretch as far as is comfortable. Also, you can place a pillow under your head for more comfort.

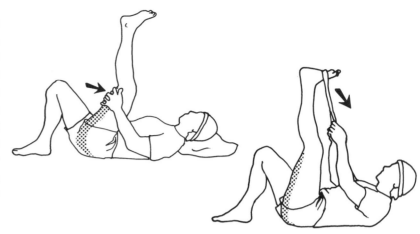

To Stretch the Groin Area

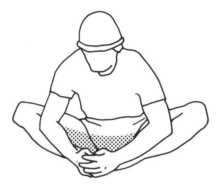 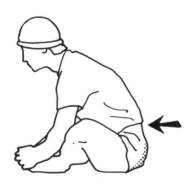

Put the soles of your feet together and hold onto your toes. Gently pull yourself forward, bending from the hips until you feel a good stretch in your groin. You may also feel a stretch in the back. Hold for 20 seconds. Do not make the initial movement for this stretch from your head and shoulders. Move from the hips (*see p. 16, Getting Started*). Try to get your elbows on the outside of your legs so you are stable and balanced. Contract your abdominal muscles mildly as you lean forward; this will increase your forward flexibility.

Remember—no bouncing when you stretch. Find a place that is fairly comfortable, one that allows you to stretch and relax at the same time.

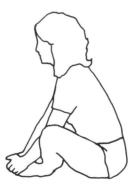 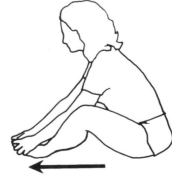

If you have any trouble bending forward, your heels may be too close to your groin area.

If so, move your feet farther out in front of you. This will allow you to move forward from your hips.

Variations if You Are Tight in the Groin Area

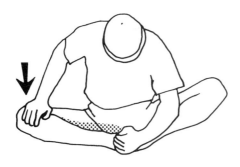

Hold onto your feet with one hand, with your elbow on the inside of the lower leg to hold down and stabilize the leg. Now, with your other hand on the inside of your leg *(not on the knee)*, gently push your leg downward to isolate and stretch this side of the groin. If you are tight in the groin area, this is a good isolation stretch that will limber up your groin and allow your knees to fall more naturally downward. Do both sides. Hold for 10–15 seconds.

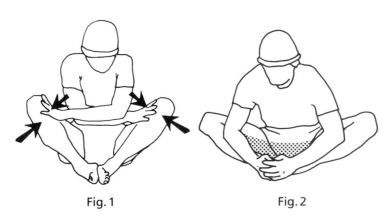

Fig. 1   Fig. 2

PNF Technique: *Contract—Relax—Stretch.* With your hands supplying slight resistance on the insides of opposite thighs, try to bring your knees together just enough to contract the muscles in the groin *(fig. 1)*. Hold this stabilized tension for 4–5 seconds, then relax and stretch the groin as in the preceding stretches *(fig. 2)*. This will help relax a tight groin area. This technique of contract-relax-stretch is valuable for athletes with groin problems.

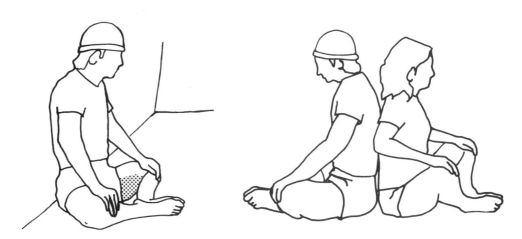

Another way to stretch tight groin muscles is to sit against a wall or couch: something that will provide support. With your back straight and the soles of your feet together, use your hands to push gently down on the inside of your thighs (not *on* the knees, just above them). Push gently until you get a good, even stretch. Relax and hold for 20–30 seconds.

It is also possible to do this stretch with a partner. Sit back-to-back for stability.

If you have trouble sitting cross-legged, these groin stretches will start to make that position easier for you.

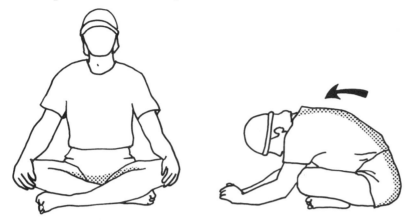

To stretch the back and inside of the legs, sit in a crossed-leg position and then lean forward until you feel a good comfortable stretch. Get your elbows out in front of you if you can. Hold and relax. This is a simple stretch for most people and really feels good in the lower back. Do not hold your breath. Stretch for 15–20 seconds.

Variation: Move your upper body over your knee instead of straight ahead. This is good for your hips. Think of bending from the hips.

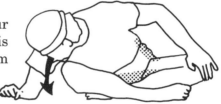

The Spinal Twist

The spinal twist is good for the upper back, lower back, side of hips, and rib cage. It will improve your ability to turn to the side or look behind you without having to turn your entire body.

Sit with your right leg straight. Bend your left leg, cross your left foot over and to the outside of your right knee. Then bend your right elbow and rest it on the outside of your upper left thigh just above the knee. Use your elbow to keep this leg stationary with controlled pressure to the inside.

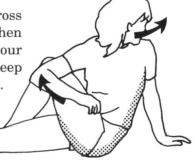

Now, with your left hand resting behind you, exhale slowly and turn your head to look over your left shoulder; at the same time rotate your upper body toward your left hand and arm. As you turn your upper body, think of turning your hips in the same direction (though your hips won't move because your right elbow is keeping the left leg stationary). This should give you a stretch in your lower back and side of hip. Hold for 10–15 seconds. Do both sides.

Breathing:
• Deep
• Relaxed
• Rhythmic

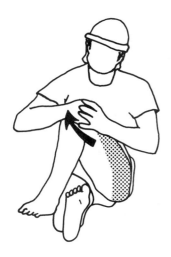

Variation: Pull your knee across your body toward your opposite shoulder until you feel an easy stretch on the side of the hip. Hold for 20–30 seconds. Do both sides.

People tend to spend more time on the first leg, arm, or area they stretch, and they usually will stretch their "easy" or more flexible side first. Thus more time is spent on the "good" side and less on the "bad" side. To remedy this, stretch your tight side first. This will help even out your overall flexibility.

SUMMARY OF STRETCHES FOR LOWER BACK, HIPS, GROIN, AND HAMSTRINGS

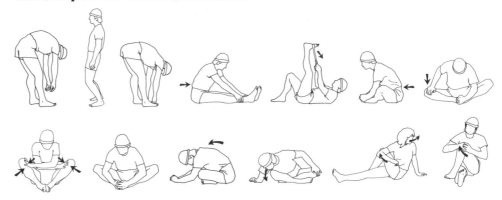

You can do these stretches, in this order, as a routine.

At this time let's go over some of the basic techniques of stretching:

- Don't stretch too far, especially in the beginning. Get a slight stretch and increase it after you feel yourself relax.

- Hold a stretch in a comfortable position; the stretch tension should subside as you hold it. No drastic static stretches.

- Breathe slowly, deeply, and naturally—exhale as you bend forward. Do not stretch to a point where you cannot breathe normally.

- Do not bounce. Bouncing tightens the very muscles you are trying to stretch.

- *Think about the area being stretched.* Feel the stretch. If the tension becomes greater as you stretch, you are overdoing it. Ease off into a more comfortable position.

- Don't focus on flexibility. Just learn to stretch properly and flexibility will come with time. (Flexibility is only one of the many by-products of stretching.)

Other things to be aware of:

- We are different every day. Some days we are tighter, other days looser.

- Drink plenty of water. Your muscles stretch more easily when your body is properly hydrated.

- You can control what you feel by what you do.

- Regularity is one of the most important factors in stretching. Stretch regularly and you will naturally want to become more active and fit.

- Don't compare yourself with others. Even if you are tight or inflexible, don't let this stop you from stretching and improving yourself.

- Proper stretching means stretching within your own limits, being relaxed, and not making comparisons with what other people can do.

- Stretching keeps your body ready for movement.

- Stretch whenever you feel like it. It will always make you feel good.

Stretches for the Back, Hips, and Legs

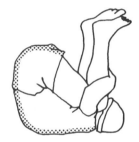

Lie on your back and pull your left leg toward your chest. Keep the back of your head on the mat if possible, but don't strain. If you can't do it with your head down, use a small pillow under your head. Keep the other leg as straight as possible, without locking your knee. Hold for 30 seconds. Do both sides. This will slowly loosen up the back muscles and hamstrings.

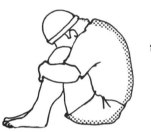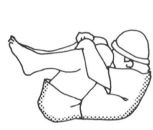

Spinal Roll: Don't do this stretch on a hard surface; use a mat or rug. In a sitting position hold your knees with your hands and pull them to your chest. Gently roll up and down your spine, keeping your chin down toward your chest. This will further stretch the muscles along the spine.

Try to roll evenly and with control. Roll back and forth 4–8 times or until you feel your back start to limber up. Do not rush.

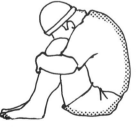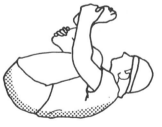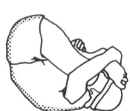

Spinal Roll with Crossed Legs: Next is the spinal roll with lower legs crossed. Begin your roll in the same sitting position as for the previous spinal roll. As you roll backwards, cross your lower legs and, at the same time, pull your feet (from the outside) toward your chest. Then, release your feet as you roll up to a sitting position with your feet together and uncrossed. (Always start each roll with the legs uncrossed.)

On each repetition, alternate the crossing of your lower legs so that, with the pull-down phase of the roll, the lower back will be stretched evenly on both sides. Do 6–8 repetitions.

> **Caution:** *If your back is extremely tight, do not stretch it too much at the beginning.* Work on the technique and balance; always pull your legs toward your chest with a constant, easy pull. Work slow and easy, concentrating on relaxing. Be patient.

Take your time in stretching your back. Do not rush through the stretches. Concentrate on relaxing in every stretch that you do. Find a stretch tension that feels good. Do not torture yourself.

> **Be careful:** If you have a neck (cervical) or lower back problem, be very careful with these stretches and variations. These are difficult stretches for many people. If you find them unpleasant, don't do them.

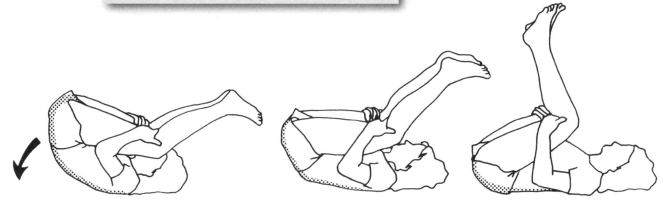

With legs in a moderate overhead position, roll down slowly, trying to roll on each vertebra, one at a time. At first you will probably come down fast, but if you practice, your back will limber up so you will be able to lower yourself slowly, vertebra after vertebra.

Put your hands directly behind your knees and *keep your knees bent* as you roll down. Use your arms and hands to hold your legs still. This will give you greater control of the speed at which you lower yourself. Keep your head on the floor. You may need to tilt your head slightly upward for balance as you roll downward.

Rolling out of the legs-overhead position slowly like this is a good way to find out exactly what part of your back is the tightest. The part or parts of your back that are the hardest to lower *slowly* are the tightest. But you can stretch the tightness and inflexibility out of the spine if you spend a little time working on it gently every day.

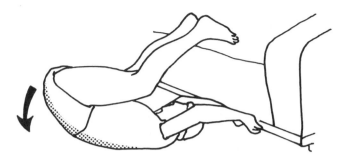

To gain more control over the stretch in your back when lowering your legs, place your arms over your head and hold onto something that is stable such as a heavy piece of furniture. Now, with a slight bend in your arms and bent knees, *slowly* lower yourself one vertebra at a time. By holding onto something with your hands you are able to stretch the back more fully. Do this slowly and under control.

Do not overdo things, but instead, *gradually* develop your physical well-being.

Stretching with legs in a moderate overhead position is good for stretching the back and helps in the circulation of blood from the lower limbs to the upper body.

The Squat: Many of us get tired in the lower back from hours of standing and sitting. One position that helps to reduce this tension is the squat.

Be careful: I believe that the squat is one of our most natural positions. However, due to particular knee problems, some people cannot and should not squat. Always check with a qualified professional if you have any concerns about what your body is capable of.

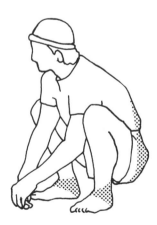

From a standing position, squat down with your feet flat and toes pointed out at approximately 15° angles. Your heels should be 4–12 inches apart, depending on how limber you are, or as you become familiar with stretching, depending on exactly what parts of your body you want to stretch. The squat stretches the knees, back, ankles, Achilles tendon areas, and deep groin. Keep your knees to the outside of your shoulders, directly above the big toes. Hold comfortably for 10–15 seconds. For many people this will be easy, for others very difficult.

Variations: At first there may be a problem with balance, such as falling backwards because of tight ankles and tight Achilles tendons. If you are unable to squat as shown above, there are other ways to learn this position.

Try the squat on the downward slant of a driveway or hillside

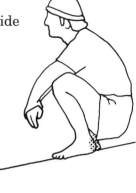

or by leaning your back against a wall.

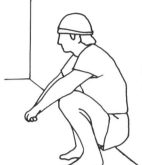

You can use a fence or pole for balance.

After you have done it for a while, the squat becomes a very comfortable position and helps relieve tightness in the lower back. Now return to a standing position as shown on the opposite page.

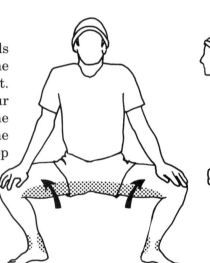

Variations: From a standing position, place your hands slightly to the inside of your upper legs, just above the knees. Your feet should be at least shoulder-width apart. Slowly lower your hips downward as you gently push your upper legs outward until you feel a mild stretch in the groin area. Hold for 15 seconds. This also stretches the ankles and Achilles tendon area. Don't let your hips drop below your knees.

Be careful if you have had any knee problems. If pain is present, discontinue this stretch.

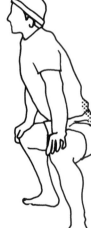

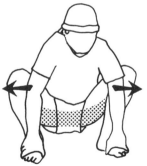

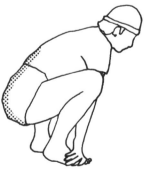

To increase the stretch in the groin from the squat position, put your elbows on the inside of your knees, gently push outward with both elbows as you bend slightly forward from your hips. Your thumbs should be on the inside of your feet, with your fingers along the outside of the feet. Hold for 15 seconds. Do not overstretch. If you have trouble balancing, elevate your heels slightly.

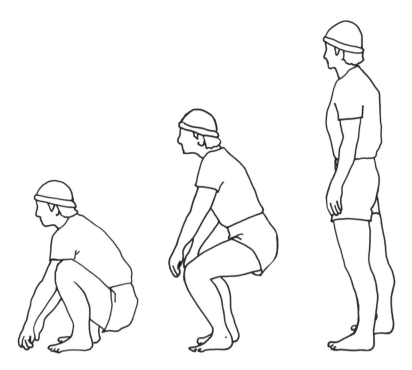

To stand up from the squat position, pull your chin in slightly and rise straight up *with your quadriceps doing all the work and your back straight.* Do not dip your head forward as you stand up; this puts too much pressure on your lower back and neck.

SUMMARY OF STRETCHES FOR THE BACK, HIPS, AND LEGS

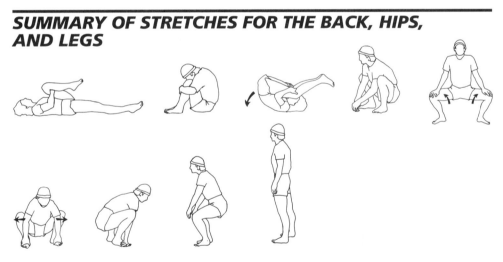

You can do these stretches, in this order, as a routine for your back.

Holding the right stretch tensions for a period of time allows the body to adapt to these new positions. Soon the area being stretched will adapt to the slight tension and your body will be able to assume the new positions without the tightness formerly felt.

Elevating Your Feet

Elevation of the feet before and after activity is a great way to revitalize your legs. It helps keep the legs light with plenty of consistent energy for everyday living and activity. It's a wonderful way to rest and relax tired feet, especially if you have been standing all day. It helps the entire body feel good. And it's a simple way to help prevent or relieve varicose veins. I recommend elevating the feet at least twice a day for 2–3 minutes or longer for revitalization and relaxation.

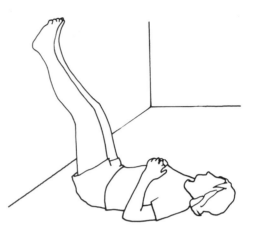

Lying on the floor and resting your feet against a wall is a simple way to elevate your feet. Keep your lower back flat. Your butt should be at least 3 inches from the wall If there isn't a wall close by, you can elevate your feet from the legs-overhead position or simply put a few pillows under your feet to raise them above your heart. At first, elevate your feet for only about one minute, gradually increasing the time. If your feet start to go to sleep, roll over on your side and then sit up. (See p. 20 for the proper way to sit up from this position.) *Don't get up quickly after elevating your feet* or you may get a light-headed feeling.

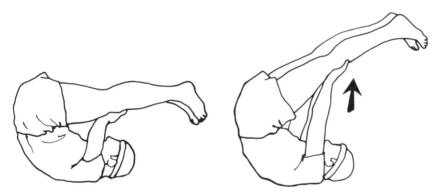

Put the palms of your hands on your knees with fingers pointed toward your toes. Straighten your arms. If you relax at the hips, your arms will take care of the weight of your legs. This is a very relaxing position. In hatha yoga it is called the "pose of tranquility." There is a balancing point, at the back of your head and the top of the spine when you are in this position. The balance is difficult to find but not as hard as it might seem at first. Give it at least 10–12 good tries. A little practice makes it simple.

Be careful doing this if you have any problem with your upper back or neck.

> We may know that stretching and regular exercising are beneficial, but knowledge alone is not enough. *Doing* is what is important, for what good is knowledge if we do not use it to live more fully?

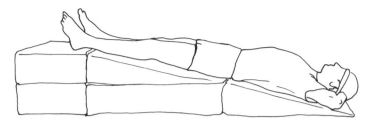

The BodySlant®: A great way to elevate your feet and stretch is to lie on a BodySlant. Don't do any exercises on the BodySlant, just lie there and relax for about 5 minutes, gradually increasing the time to 15–20 minutes. Placing your hands on your chest or stomach will decrease the arch in your lower back.

This is a good position for pulling in your stomach and being thin. The internal organs will gradually fall back into a normal position. For people who want to look and feel thin, the BodySlant is excellent.

When getting up from the BodySlant, sit up for 2–3 minutes before you stand. You should get up slowly from all positions with feet elevated so you don't become dizzy.

Stretching on the BodySlant

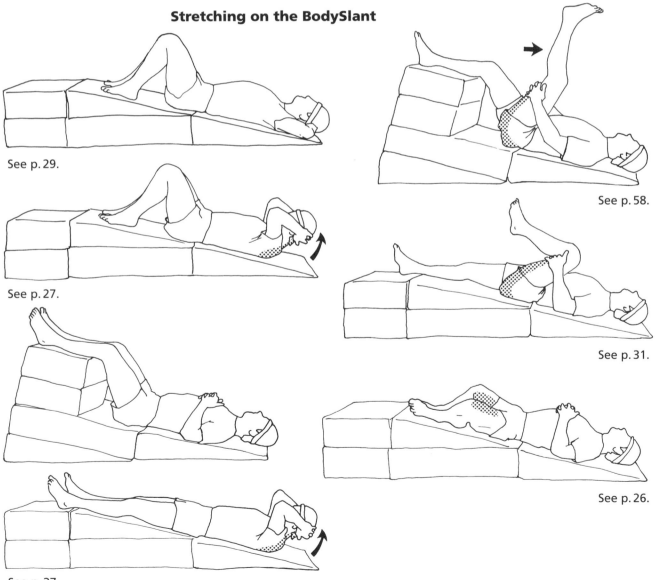

See p. 29.

See p. 27.

See p. 27.

See p. 58.

See p. 31.

See p. 26.

SUMMARY OF STRETCHES FOR ELEVATING YOUR FEET

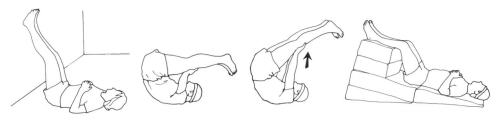

Standing Stretches for Legs and Hips

This series of stretches will help your walking or running. It will give flexibility and energy to your legs. All these stretches can be done while standing.

If possible, hold onto something for balance. Lift your left foot up off the floor and rotate your foot and ankle 10–12 times clockwise, then 10–12 times counterclockwise. Repeat for right foot and ankle. This activates circulation in the legs.

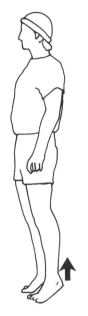

PNF Technique: Contract—Relax—Stretch. Before stretching your calves, stand on your toes for 3–4 seconds to contract your calves. Then use the following calf stretch. This should make it easier.

To stretch your calf, stand a little way from a solid support and lean on it with your forearms, head resting on hands. Bend one leg and place your foot on the ground in front of you, with the other leg straight behind. Slowly move your hips forward, keeping your lower back flat. Be sure to keep the heel of the straight leg on the ground, with toes pointed straight ahead or slightly turned in. Hold an easy stretch for 10–15 seconds. Do not bounce. Now stretch other leg. *Also see p. 15,* Getting Started.

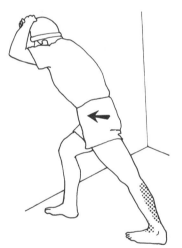

To create a stretch for the *soleus* and Achilles tendon area, lower your hips downward as you bend your knee slightly. Be sure to keep your back flat. Your back foot should be slightly toed-in or straight ahead during the stretch. Keep your heel down. This stretch is good for developing ankle flexibility. Hold for 10 seconds. The Achilles tendon area needs only a *slight feeling of stretch.*

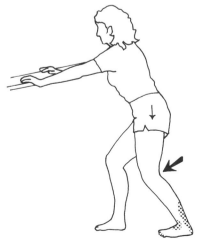

The Achilles tendon area and ankle may be stretched another way. Place your left foot against a wall, with your ankle flexed and toes up as shown in the illustration. Move your upper body forward until you feel a mild stretch tension in the Achilles tendon area. Hold for 8–10 seconds. This also stretches the bottom of your foot and toes.

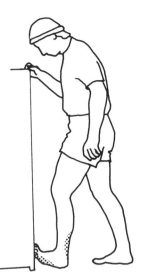

To stretch the outside of the hip, start from the same position as in the calf stretch. Stretch the right side of your hip by turning your right hip slightly to the inside. Project the side of your right hip to the side as you lean your shoulders very slightly in the opposite direction of your hips. Hold an even stretch for 10–15 seconds. Do both sides. Keep the foot of your back leg pointed straight ahead with the heel flat on ground.

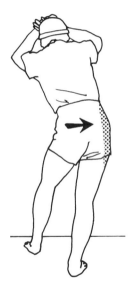

Lifelong Fitness Could Start in School

In the old days, high school students spent many hours in PE classes, learning only games and sports. If stretching was taught at all, it was the bouncing, "no pain—no gain" approach. These days a new generation of teachers has the opportunity to teach students how to take care of themselves: to stretch properly, to eat right, to make exercise a natural component of a healthy lifestyle. It would be great if kids could come out of school with a positive attitude toward staying healthy for the rest of their lives.

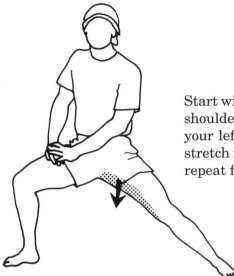

Start with your feet pointed straight ahead and a little more than shoulder-width apart. Bend your right knee slightly and move your left hip downward toward the right knee. This gives you a stretch in left inner thigh (left groin). Hold for 10–15 seconds and repeat for your right thigh.

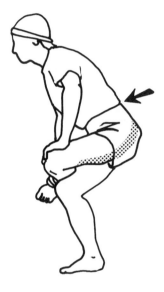

Stand on one foot with your knee slightly flexed and place the outside of the opposite leg just above your knee. Put one hand on the inside of your ankle and the other on your thigh. Now bend your knee a little more as you move your chest forward over the bent leg. This will test your balance. Hold a mild stretch for 10 seconds. Do both sides. This stretches the outside of the hip (*piriformis* area). Do not hold your breath.

Hold onto something and pull your knee toward your chest. Do not lean forward at the waist or hips. This gently stretches your upper hamstrings, butt, and hips. The foot on the ground should be pointed straight ahead, with the knee slightly bent (1 inch). Hold an easy stretch for 10–15 seconds. Do both legs.

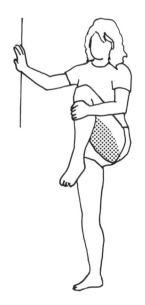

Place the ball of your foot up on a secure support of some kind (wall, fence, table). Keep the standing leg pointed straight ahead. Now bend the knee of the raised leg as you move your hips forward. This should stretch your groin, hamstrings, and front of hip. Hold for 10–15 seconds. Do both sides. If you can, for balance and control, use your hands to hold onto the support. This stretch will make it easier to lift your knees.

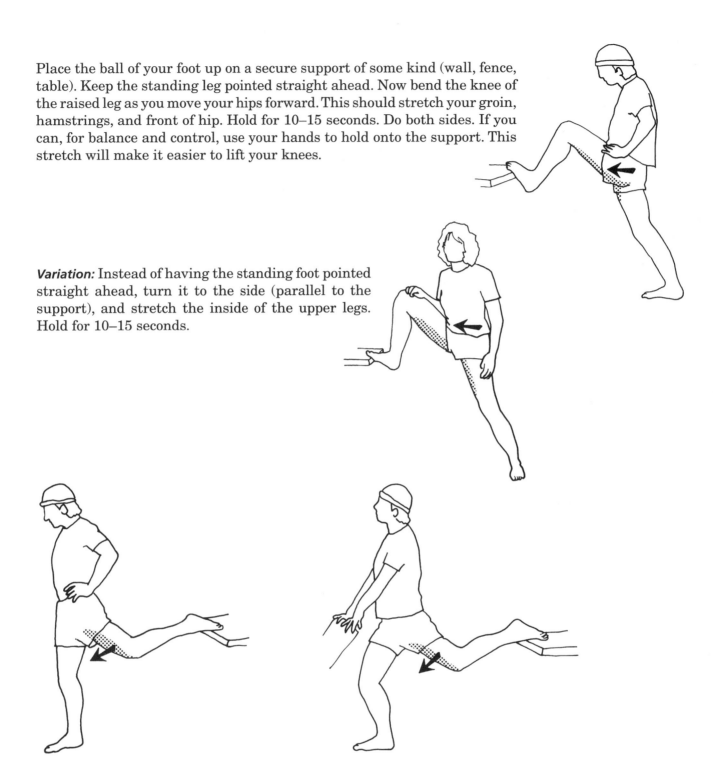

Variation: Instead of having the standing foot pointed straight ahead, turn it to the side (parallel to the support), and stretch the inside of the upper legs. Hold for 10–15 seconds.

Extend your foot behind you, placing the top of your foot on a table, fence, or bar at a comfortable height. Think of pulling your leg through (moving your leg forward) from the front of your hip to create a stretch for the front of the hip and quadriceps. Flex your butt (*gluteus*) muscles as you do this stretch. Keep the standing knee slightly bent (1 inch) and the upper body vertical. The foot on the ground should be pointed straight ahead. You can change the stretch by slightly bending the knee of the supporting leg a little more. Hold an easy stretch for 10–15 seconds. Through relaxed practice, learn to feel balanced and comfortable in this stretch. Breathe. Use a chair or something for balance if necessary.

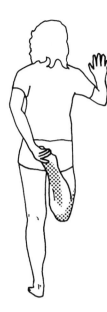

To stretch the quads and knee, hold the top of your *right* foot with your left hand and gently pull your heel toward your buttocks. The knee bends at a natural angle when you hold your foot with the opposite hand. This is good to use in knee rehabilitation and with problem knees. Hold up to 10–20 seconds for each leg.

Variation: This stretch can also be done lying on your stomach. Be sure to stretch without pain. Reach behind you with your hand and hold the top of your opposite foot between the ankle joint and toes. Gently pull your heel toward the middle of your buttocks. Hold for 10–15 seconds.

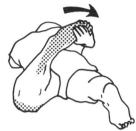

Important note: If you have knee problems, be very careful with these stretches.

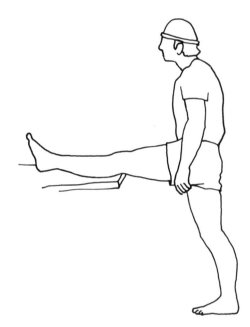

Remember to stretch under control. Start in a place that is fairly easy and go from there. Improvement will occur faster if you go from an easy stretch to a developmental stretch. Let yourself limber up slowly. Remember, straining will keep you from fully realizing the many benefits of stretching.

Place the back of your lower leg on a table or ledge that is about waist high or at a comfortable height. The leg on the ground should be slightly bent at the knee (1 inch), with your foot pointed forward as in a proper running or walking position.

Be careful to not overstretch in this position. Overstretching can put too much stress on the back of the knee, especially if the lower leg is not supported fully.

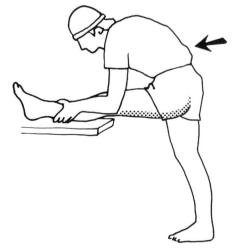

Now, while looking straight ahead, slowly bend forward at the hips until you feel a good stretch in the back of the raised leg. Hold for 10–15 seconds and relax. Find the easy stretch, relax, and then increase it slightly. This is very good for running or walking.

Keep your knees slightly flexed with all these leg-up stretches.

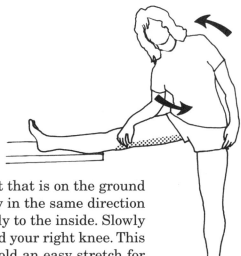

To stretch the inside of your raised leg, turn the foot that is on the ground so it is parallel to the support. Face your upper body in the same direction as your standing foot and turn your right hip slightly to the inside. Slowly bend sideways with your right shoulder going toward your right knee. This should stretch the inside of your upper right leg. Hold an easy stretch for 10–15 seconds. Be sure to keep the knee of the standing leg slightly bent. Repeat for the other leg.

Variation: To change the stretch, use your right hand to pull your left hand and arm up and over your head. This is good for the sides of your upper body and the inside of your raised leg. Keep the knee of the standing leg slightly bent. Hold an easy stretch for 10–15 seconds. Do both sides. Feel the difference in each side. To do this stretch you must be fairly flexible.

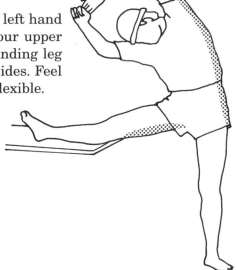

Remember: Take care with these more difficult stretches, which require balance, strength, and a certain amount of flexibility.

To change the stretch, bend at the waist toward the foot on the ground. The raised leg should remain straight but will turn to the inside as you bend over. This stretches the hamstrings of the supporting leg. The knee of that leg should be slightly bent (1 inch) during the stretch. Hold an easy stretch for 10–15 seconds. Do not hold your breath.

If you want to stretch the groin area of the raised leg, bend the knee of the supporting leg and keep the raised leg straight. If you can, rest your hands on the ground to give you added balance. Hold an easy stretch for 10–15 seconds.

SUMMARY OF STANDING STRETCHES FOR LEGS AND HIPS

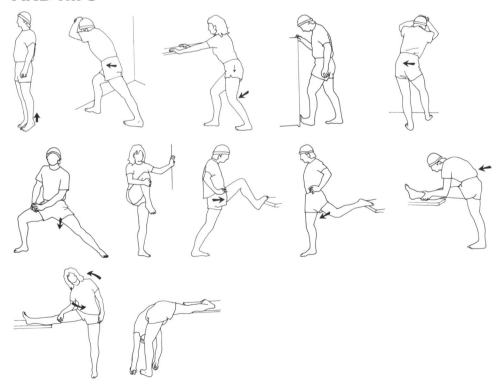

You can do these stretches, in this order, as a routine for the legs and hips.

Avoid creeping *rigor mortis*: It is important to maintain good flexibility throughout our lives, so that as we get older we can avoid the problems that go with stiff joints, tight muscles, and bad posture. One of the striking characteristics of aging is the loss of range of motion, and stretching is perhaps the single most important thing you can do to keep your body limber.

Standing Stretches for the Upper Body

These next two stretches are excellent for stretching the muscles along your side from your arm to your hips. They are done standing, so you can do them at any time, anywhere. Remember to keep your knees slightly bent (flexed) for better balance and to protect your lower back.

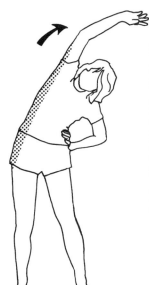

Stand with your feet about shoulder-width apart and toes pointed straight ahead. With knees slightly bent (1 inch), place one hand on your hip for support while you extend your other arm up and over your head. Now slowly bend at your waist to the side, toward the hand on your hip. Move slowly; feel a good stretch. Hold for 10–15 seconds and relax. Gradually increase the amount of time you are able to hold the stretch. Always come out of a stretch slowly and under control. No quick or jerky movements. Breathe and relax.

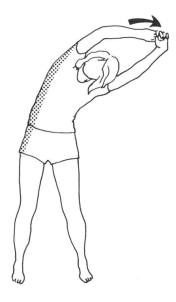

Instead of using your hand on your hip for support, extend both arms overhead. Grasp your right hand with your left hand and bend slowly to the left, using your left arm to gently pull the right arm over the head and down toward the ground.

By using one arm to pull the other you can increase the stretch along your sides and along the spine. *Do not overstretch.* Hold an easy stretch for 8–10 seconds.

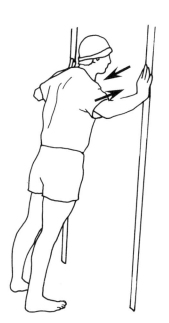
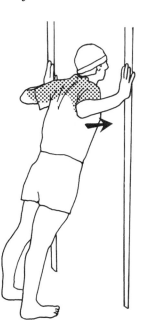

PNF Technique: *Contract—Relax—Stretch.* Stand behind a doorway. With your hands on the door jambs a little above shoulder height, with arms bent, push yourself back by straightening your arms, as in a push-up. Do 3–5 repetitions of this exercise, then relax and slowly let your upper body go toward the doorway to stretch the front of your shoulders and chest. Hold for 15–20 seconds at a comfortable tension.

This stretch for the upper body stretches the muscles laterally along the spine.

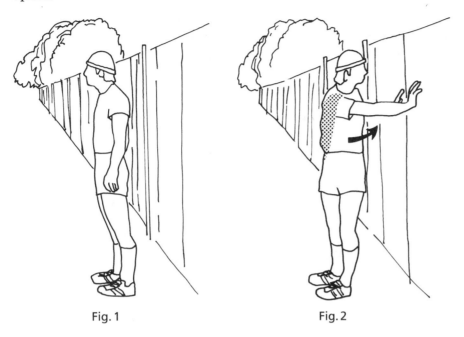

Fig. 1   Fig. 2

Stand about 12–24 inches away from a fence or wall with your back toward it *(fig. 1)*. With your feet about shoulder-width apart and toes pointed straight ahead, slowly turn your upper body around until you can easily place your hands on the fence or wall at about shoulder height *(fig. 2)*. Turn in one direction and touch the wall, return to the starting position, and then turn in the opposite direction and touch the wall. Do not force yourself to turn any farther than is fairly comfortable. If you have a knee problem, do this stretch very slowly and cautiously. Stop if there is pain. Be relaxed and do not overstretch. Hold for 10–15 seconds. Keep knees slightly bent (1 inch). Do not hold your breath. Stretch the other side.

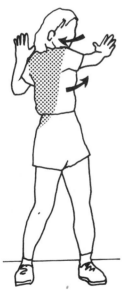

Variation: To change the stretch, turn your head and look over your right shoulder. Try to keep your hips facing forward and parallel to the fence. Hold an easy stretch for 10 seconds. Do both sides.

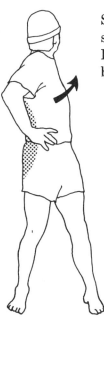

Start with your hands on your hips, feet pointed straight ahead, knees slightly bent. Rotate hips to the left as you look over your left shoulder. Hold an easy stretch for 10 seconds. Stretch each side twice. Be relaxed and breathe easily. This is a good stretch for lower back, hips, and upper body.

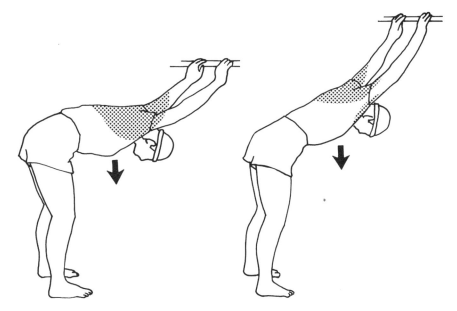

Another good upper body and back stretch is to place both hands shoulder-width apart on a fence or ledge (or the top of refrigerator or filing cabinet) and let your upper body drop down as you keep your knees slightly bent (1 inch). Your hips should be directly above your feet, your breathing rhythmical.

Now, bend your knees just a bit more and feel the stretch change. Place your hands at different heights to change the area of the stretch. After you become familiar with this stretch it is possible to really stretch the spine. Great to do if you have been slumping in the upper back and shoulders all day. This will take some of the kinks out of a tired upper back. Find a stretch that you can hold for at least 20 seconds. Bend your knees when coming out of this stretch.

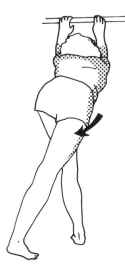

Variation: To increase and change the area of the stretch in another way, bring one leg behind and across the midline of your body as you lean in the opposite direction. This will stretch those hard-to-reach areas of the upper body. Hold for 10 seconds. Do both sides.

I find these arm and shoulder stretches to be very good before and after running. They allow for a relaxed upper body and a freer arm swing. They are also good to do during weight training workouts or as a warm-up for any upper body activity such as tennis, baseball, handball, etc.

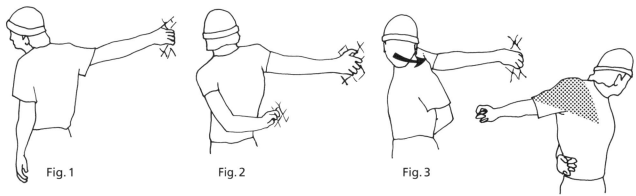

Fig. 1   Fig. 2   Fig. 3

View from the other side of the fence

This stretch is for the front of the shoulders and arms. You need a chain-linked fence, doorway, or wall. Face the wall or press against it with your right hand at shoulder level *(fig. 1)*. Next, bring your other arm around your back and grab the wall (or whatever you are using) as in fig. 2. Now, look over your left shoulder in the direction of your right hand. Keep your shoulder close to the wall as you slowly turn your head *(fig. 3)*. Trying to look at your right hand behind you gives you a stretch in the front of the shoulders.

Stretch the other side. Do it slowly and under control. The feeling of a good stretch is what is important, *not how far you can stretch.*

Variation: From the previous position, stretch your arm and shoulder at various angles. Each angle will stretch the arm and shoulder differently. Hold for 10 seconds.

Here is another stretch you can do while using a chain-linked fence or wall for support and balance.

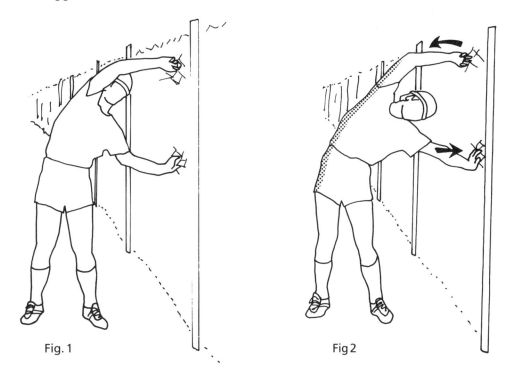

Fig. 1

Fig 2

Hold onto the fence at about waist-high with your left hand. Now reach over your head with your right arm and grab the fence with your right hand. Your left arm will be slightly bent with the right arm extended *(fig. 1)*. Keep knees slightly bent (1 inch).

To stretch your waistline and sides, straighten your left arm and pull over with your (upper) right arm *(fig. 2)*. Hold for 10 seconds. Do both sides.

> Slowly go into each stretch and slowly come out of each stretch. Do not bob, jerk, or bounce. Keep your stretching fluid and under control.

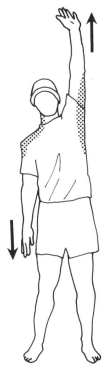

Reach in opposite directions with your arms while standing. Hold for 10 seconds each side. Keep your jaw relaxed and breathe rhythmically. This is an excellent stretch for upper body tension. It stretches the sides of the upper body, shoulders, and arms.

SUMMARY OF STANDING STRETCHES FOR THE UPPER BODY

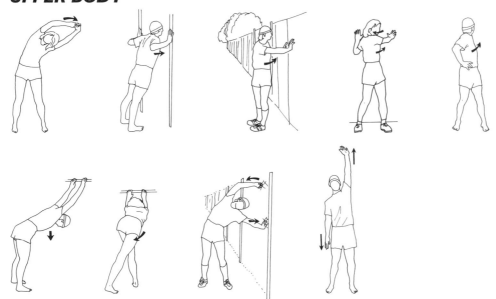

You can do these stretches, in this order, as a routine for the upper body.

Stretching on a Chin-up Bar

With the help of gravity, it is possible to get a fine stretch on a chin bar.

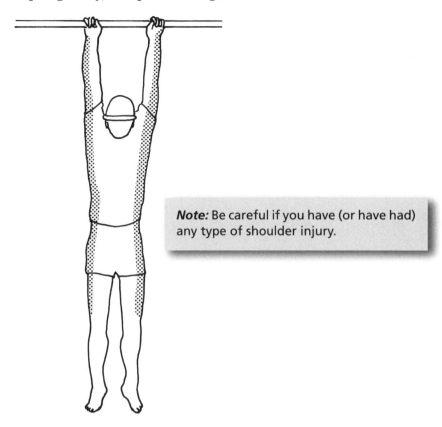

Note: Be careful if you have (or have had) any type of shoulder injury.

Hold onto the bar with both hands, relax your chin forward as you hang, with feet off the ground. A great stretch for the upper body. Begin holding for 5 seconds, gradually increasing to at least 30 seconds. A strong grip will make this stretch easier.

Enjoy stretching by the way it feels. If you torture yourself with drastic tensions in an attempt to get more flexible, you deprive yourself of the true benefits of stretching. If you stretch correctly, you'll find the more you stretch, the easier it becomes, and the easier you stretch, the more you will naturally enjoy it.

Stretches for the Upper Body Using a Towel

Most of us have a towel in our hands at least once a day. A towel or elastic cord can aid in stretching the arms, shoulders, and chest.

Hold the towel near both ends so that you can move it, with straight arms, up and over your head and down behind your back. Do not strain or force it. Your hands should be far enough apart to allow for relatively free movement up and over your head and down behind your back. Breathe slowly. Do not hold your breath.

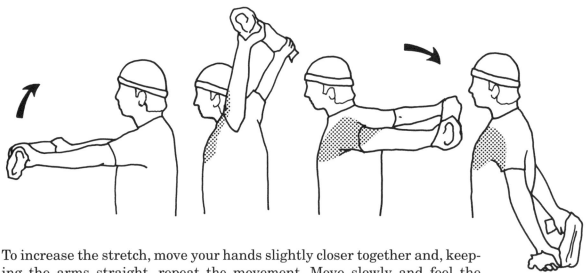

To increase the stretch, move your hands slightly closer together and, keeping the arms straight, repeat the movement. Move slowly and feel the stretch. Do not overstretch. If you are unable to go through the full movement of up, over, and behind while keeping your arms straight, then your hands are too close together. Move them farther apart.

You can hold the stretch at any place during this movement. This will isolate and add more of a stretch to the muscles of that particular area. For example, if your chest is tight and sore, it is possible to isolate the stretch there by holding the towel at shoulder level with arms straight behind you, as shown above. Hold for 10–15 seconds.

> Stretching is not a contest. You needn't compare yourself with others, because we are all different. Moreover, each day we are different: some days we are more limber than others. Stretch comfortably, within your limits, and you will begin to feel the flow of energy that comes from proper stretching.

Here is another series of stretches using a towel.

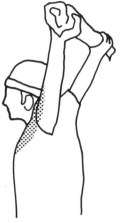 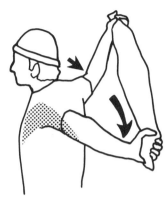

Bring the towel overhead, keeping your arms straight.

Lower the left arm back and behind you at shoulder level as your right arm bends to approximately a 90° angle.

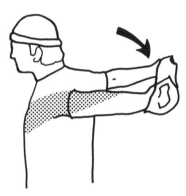 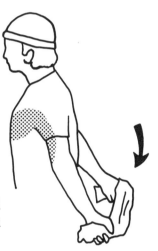

Now straighten the right arm out to the same level as the left arm and then simultaneously move both arms downward.

This can he done slowly, in one complete movement, or you can stop at any point to increase the stretch in that particular area. Do this completed movement toward the other side by lowering your right arm first.

As you become more flexible, you will be able to hold the towel with your hands closer together. But again, do not strain.

I think that limberness in the shoulders and arms really helps tennis, running, walking, and of course swimming (to name only a few activities for which you need this flexibility). Stretching the chest area reduces muscle tension and tightness and increases circulation and ease of breathing. It is actually very simple to stretch and keep the upper body limber, if you do it *regularly.*

Note: Be careful if you have (or have had) any type of shoulder injury. Proceed slowly and discontinue if there is pain.

A Series of Stretches for Hands, Wrists, and Forearms (Sitting or Standing)

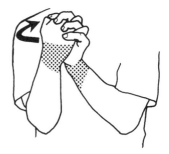

First, interlace your fingers in front of you and rotate your hands and wrists clockwise 10 times.

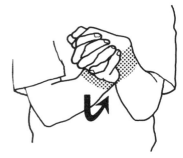

Repeat counterclockwise 10 times. This will improve the flexibility of your hands and wrists and provide a slight warm-up.

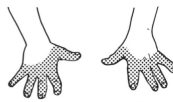

Then separate and straighten your fingers until the tension of a stretch is felt. Hold for 10 seconds, then relax.

Next, bend your fingers at the knuckles and hold for 10 seconds. Then relax.

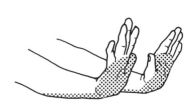

Now, with your arms straight out in front of you, bend your wrists with fingers pointing upwards. This will stretch the back of your forearms. Hold for 10–12 seconds. Do twice.

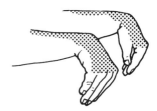

Then bend your wrist with your fingers pointing downwards to stretch the top of your forearms. Hold for 10–12 seconds. Do twice.

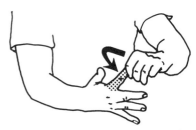

With your index finger and thumb gently hold a finger or the thumb of the opposite hand. Use your index finger and thumb to rotate each finger and thumb 5 times clockwise and counterclockwise.

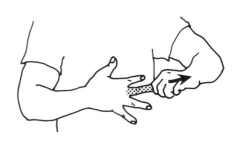

Next gently pull each finger and thumb straight out and hold for 2–3 seconds.

Now, shake your arms and hands at your sides for 10–12 seconds. Keep your jaw relaxed and let your shoulders hang downward as you shake out tension.

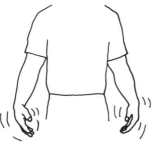

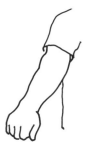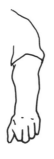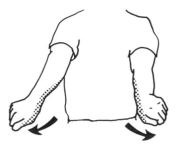

Start with your arms straight out in front of you. Slowly turn your hands to the outside (as you keep your arms straight) until a stretch is felt along the inside forearms and wrists. Hold for 5–10 seconds.

Place your hands palm-to-palm in front of you. Then, move your hands downward, keeping your palms together, until you feel a mild stretch. Keep your elbows up and even. Hold for 5–8 seconds.

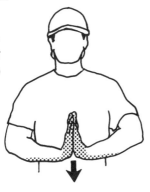

From the above stretch, rotate your palms around until they face more or less downward. Go until you feel a mild stretch. Keep your elbows up and even. Hold for 5–8 seconds.

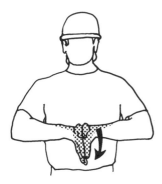

Place your hands palm-to-palm in front of you. Push one hand gently to the side until you feel a mild stretch. Keep your elbows up and even. Hold for 5–8 seconds.

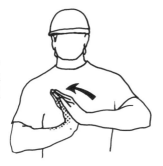

Use some or all of these stretches to counteract the problems that may come from repetitive movements, such as computer work. Use these daily, especially at work.

Sitting Stretches

A series of stretches you can do while sitting: These are good for people who work at office jobs. You can relieve tension and energize parts of your body that have become stiff from sitting.

Sitting stretches for upper body: Interlace your fingers, then straighten your arms out in front of you with palms facing out. Feel the stretch in arms and through upper part of back (shoulder blades). Hold stretch for 20 seconds. Do at least twice.

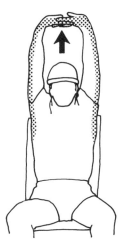

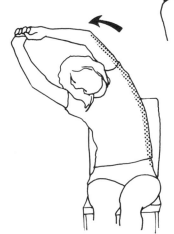

Interlace fingers, then turn palms upward above your head as you straighten your arms. Think of elongating your arms as you feel a stretch through your arms and upper sides of the rib cage. Hold only a stretch that feels good. Do three times. Hold for 10 seconds.

With arms extended overhead, hold onto the outside of your left hand with right hand and pull your left arm to the side. Keep arms as straight as comfortably possible. This will stretch the left arm and side of body and shoulder. Hold for 10 seconds. Do both sides.

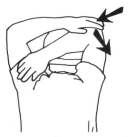

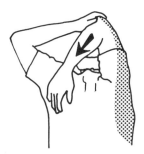

PNF Technique: Contract—Relax—Stretch. Hold your right elbow with your left hand. Move your right elbow downward as you resist this movement with your left hand (isometric contraction) for 3–4 seconds.

After relaxing a moment, gently pull your elbow over, behind your head until you feel a mild stretch in the back of your upper arm. Hold for 10–15 seconds. Repeat to other side.

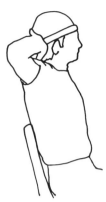

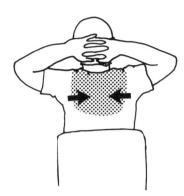

With your fingers interlaced behind your head, keep your elbows straight out to the side with your upper body in a good, aligned position. Now think of pulling your shoulder blades together to create a feeling of tension through the upper back and shoulder blades. Hold, with a feeling of releasing tension, for 4–5 seconds and then relax. Do several times. This is good to do when your shoulders and upper back are tense or tight. This is also good to do while standing.

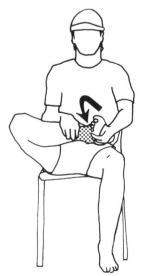

With your left hand hold your right arm just above the elbow. Now gently pull your elbow toward your left shoulder as you look over your right shoulder. Hold stretch for 10 seconds. Do both sides.

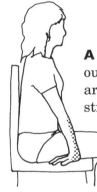

A Stretch for the Forearm: With the palm of your hand flat, thumb to the outside and fingers pointed backward, slowly lean back to stretch your forearm. Be sure to keep palms flat. Hold for 10 seconds. Do both sides. You can stretch both forearms at the same time, if you wish.

Sitting Stretches for Ankles, Side of Hip, and Lower Back

While sitting, rotate your ankles clockwise and then counterclockwise. Do one ankle at a time, 20–30 revolutions.

Hold onto your lower left leg just below the knee. Gently pull it toward your chest. To isolate a stretch in the side of your upper leg, use the left arm to pull the bent leg across and toward the opposite shoulder. Hold for 15 seconds at an easy stretch tension. Do both sides.

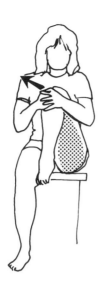

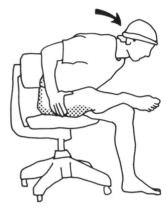

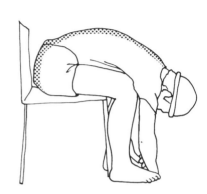

Cross you right leg over your left leg, right ankle and foot resting just to the outside of your left knee. To stretch the side of your right hip (*piriformis* area), slowly lean your upper body forward, bending from the hips until you feel a mild stretch. Hold for 10–15 seconds. Stay relaxed and breathe rhythmically. Repeat, crossing your left leg over your right leg.

Lean forward to stretch and take the pressure off your lower back. Even if you do not feel a stretch, it is still good for circulation. Hold for 15–20 seconds. Put your hands on your thighs to help push your body to an upright position.

Stretches for the Face and Neck

Raise the top of your shoulders toward your ears until you feel a slight tension in your neck and shoulder. Hold for 5 seconds, then relax shoulders downward into normal position. Do several times at the first sign of shoulder tension. It really works!

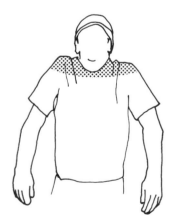

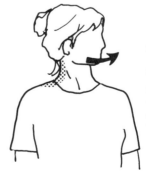

Turn your chin toward your left shoulder to create a stretch on the right side of your neck. Hold correct stretch tensions for 5–10 seconds. Stretch to each side twice. Keep your shoulders relaxed downward. Do not hold your breath.

This stretch may cause people around you to think you are a bit weird, but you often find a lot of tension in your face from frowning or squinting because of eye strain.

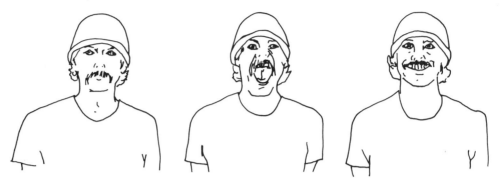

Raise your eyebrows and open your eyes as wide as possible. At the same time, open your mouth to stretch the muscles around your nose and chin and stick your tongue out. Hold this stretch for 5–10 seconds. Getting the tension out of the muscles in your face will make you smile. Do several times.

Caution: If you hear clicking or popping noises when opening your mouth, check with your dentist.

SUMMARY OF SITTING STRETCHES

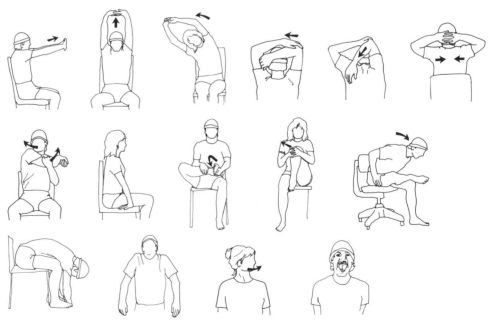

Do these sitting stretches, in this order, as a routine.

Advanced Stretches for the Legs and Groin with Feet Elevated

A wall or doorway can be useful for stretching the legs while you relax on your back. When doing these stretches think of the easy stretch, gradually increasing into the developmental stretch.

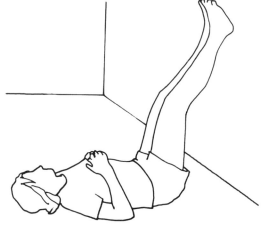

Start with your legs elevated and close together, with your butt about 3–5 inches away from the wall so that your lower back is flat and not arched or off the floor.

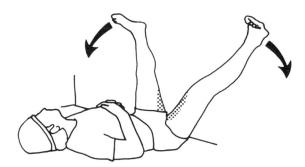

It's possible to stretch your groin from this position by slowly separating your legs, with your heels resting on the wall, until you feel an easy stretch. Hold for 30 seconds and relax. Breathe rhythmically.

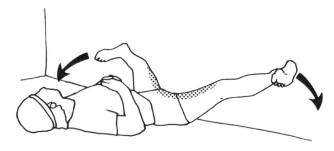

As this position becomes easier over time, you can gradually stretch further by lowering your legs. An advanced position is shown here. Do not try to copy this, but stretch within your limits. Do not strain. The wall makes it possible to hold these stretches longer in a relaxed, stable position.

Remember to keep your butt 3–5 inches from the wall. If you are too close to the wall you may feel tightness in your lower back.

Variation:

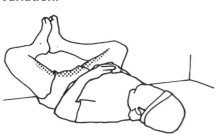

Push a little above the knee, not on the knee.

Put the soles of your feet together, resting them against the wall. Relax.

To increase the stretch, use your hands to gently push down on the inside of your thighs until you feel a good, easy stretch. Relax while you stretch. Hold for 10–15 seconds.

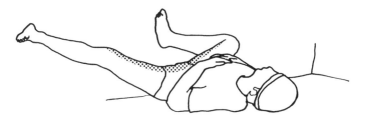

To isolate and increase the stretch in each side of the groin area, straighten one leg out. Hold each leg for 10–15 seconds.

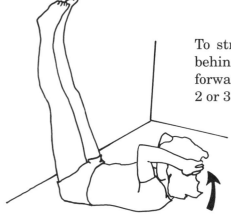

To stretch your neck from this position, interlace your fingers behind your head (at about ear level) and gently pull your head forward until you feel an easy stretch. Hold for 5 seconds. Repeat 2 or 3 times. (See p. 27 for further information on neck stretches.)

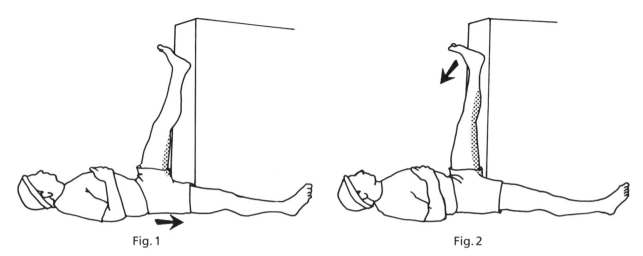

Fig. 1   Fig. 2

Here is an excellent way to stretch your hamstrings. Begin by lying on your back with your foot up on a doorway or wall and the other leg in a doorway or space where it can lie straight. To stretch the hamstrings of the leg up on the wall, move your body forward, toward the doorway, until a mild stretch is felt *(fig. 1)*. Hold for 10–15 seconds. To stretch your calf and hamstrings from this position, bring your toes toward your shin until you feel a stretch in your calf *(fig. 2)*. Hold for 10–15 seconds. Breathe easily.

SUMMARY OF ADVANCED STRETCHES FOR THE LEG AND GROIN

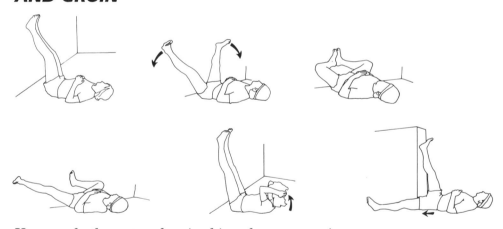

You can do these stretches, in this order, as a routine.

If you don't have much uninterrupted time available, use short periods of stretching (1–3 minutes) every three or four hours. This will help you to feel consistently good throughout the day.

Stretching the Groin and Hips with Legs Apart

The following stretches will make lateral movement easier, help maintain flexibility, and can prevent injuries. Gradually become accustomed to these stretches, which are primarily for the center of your body.

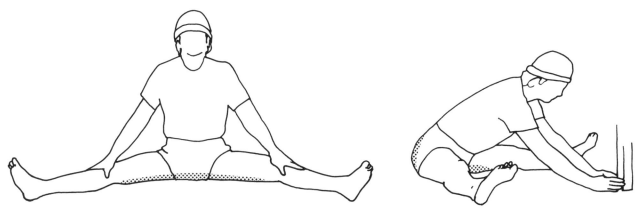

Sit with your feet a comfortable distance apart. To stretch the inside of your upper legs and hips, slowly lean forward from your hips. Be sure to keep your quadriceps relaxed and feet upright. Hold for 10–20 seconds. Keep your hands out in front of you for balance and stability or hold onto something for greater control. Breathe deeply.

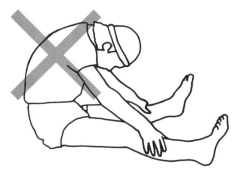

Do not lean forward with your head and shoulders. This will cause your upper back to round and put pressure on your lower back. If, when you lean forward, your lower back is rounded (causing your hips to tilt backward), it is because your hips, lower back, and hamstrings are tight. To bend from your hips correctly, you must keep your lower back straight (upright) so you can move forward from the hips (or thigh joints), and not by rounding your back.

Don't stretch to be flexible. Stretch to feel good.

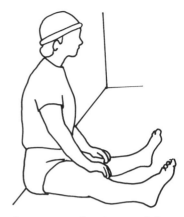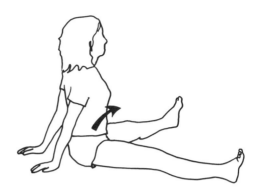

A good way to adapt your hips and lower back gradually to a proper, upright position is to sit with your lower back flat against a wall. Hold an easy stretch for 30 seconds.

Another way is to sit with your hands behind you. Using your arms as a support will help lengthen your spine as you concentrate on moving your hips slightly forward. Hold for 20 seconds.

Do not bend forward until you are able to feel comfortable doing the variations above. Get your body used to these positions before you try to stretch any further.

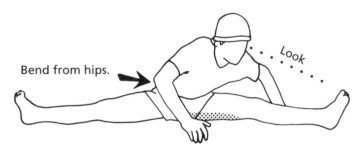

Bend from hips.   Look

Variation: To stretch your left hamstrings and the right side of your back, slowly bend forward from the hips, toward the foot of your left leg. Keep your chin in and your back straight. Hold a good stretch for at least 15–20 seconds. If necessary, use a towel. Don't look down. Look just over your toes. Stay relaxed and breathe easily.

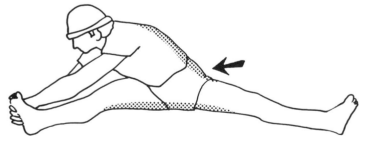

Another variation is to reach across your body with the left hand to the right foot, putting your right hand out to the right side for balance. This will increase the stretch in your hamstrings and in your back, as far up as the shoulder blades and as far down as the hips. Do this across-the-body stretch in both directions. This stretch requires good, overall flexibility. Hold for 10–15 seconds.

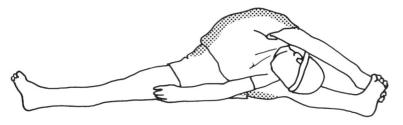

An Advanced Stretch: Reach overhead with your hand and grasp the opposite foot. Keep your other arm resting close to your body in front of you. This is a good lateral stretch for the back and legs. Hold for 15–20 seconds. Do both sides. Do not overstretch. Do not hold your breath.

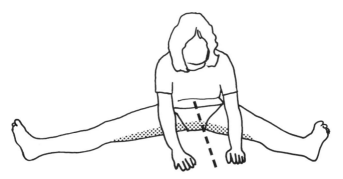

Learn to hold stretch tensions at various angles. Stretch forward, left, and right, then teach yourself to hold stretches at angles toward left of center and right of center. Use the same leg and upper body alignment as previously described. Hold for 10–15 seconds. Stretch with complete self-control.

If you feel and look tight doing these stretches, do not be discouraged. Stretch without worrying about flexibility. Then you can gradually adapt your body to these new angles with stretch tensions that feel right.

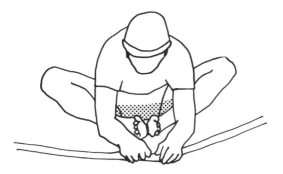

A More Advanced Groin Stretch: With the soles of your feet together, lean forward and hold onto something near the floor in front of you (this may be the edge of the mat, or the leg of a piece of furniture). Use this object to help you hold a comfortable stretch and to pull yourself forward to increase the stretch. Do not overstretch. Hold and relax for 10–20 seconds. Remember to contract your abdominals as you lean forward.

Holding onto something will stabilize your legs and make it easier to hold a stretch when you are sitting with legs apart.

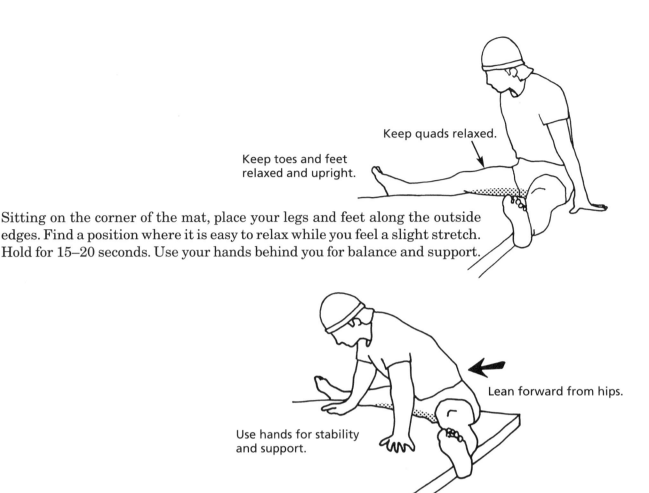

Keep quads relaxed.

Keep toes and feet relaxed and upright.

Sitting on the corner of the mat, place your legs and feet along the outside edges. Find a position where it is easy to relax while you feel a slight stretch. Hold for 15–20 seconds. Use your hands behind you for balance and support.

Lean forward from hips.

Use hands for stability and support.

To increase the stretch, move your butt and hips forward, sliding your legs down along the sides of the mat. Keep toes and feet upright. Do not let your legs turn in or out. A good stretch for limbering up groin and hips.

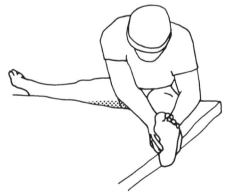

To stretch one leg at a time, sit on the corner of the mat in a comfortable position. Turn to face one foot and bend forward from the hips in that direction. Reach down with your hands and hold your leg at a point that gives you an easy stretch. Think of your chin going toward or just beyond your knee (even though it may not), as you look just above your toes. Relax. Sit up and stretch the other leg in the same way. Stretch your tightest leg first. If necessary, put a towel around the bottom of your foot to help you stretch. Hold an easy stretch for 10–20 seconds. No bouncing. This is a good stretch for the hamstrings, lower back, and hips. Breathe and relax.

Learning the Splits

This section is for a limited number of people. Unless you are training for gymnastics, dance, or need extreme flexibility (as does an ice hockey goal-keeper, or a first baseman, or a ballet dancer), the other sections in this book should handle most of your stretching needs. I'm not trying to discourage you, but for everyday living being able to do the splits is hardly necessary!

> **Note:** Be sure to do an adequate warm-up prior to these stretches. Do some easier stretches and 5–6 minutes of aerobic activity.

Forward Splits

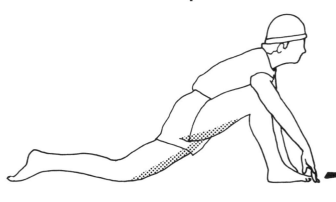

From the stretch position described on p. 51, slowly move your front foot forward until you feel a controlled stretch in the back of the legs and groin. Think of your hips going straight down. Hold for 10–20 seconds.

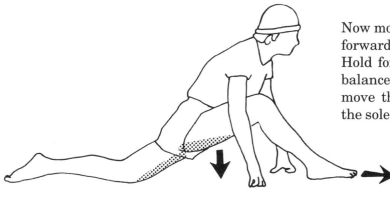

Now move your front foot a little farther forward into the developmental stretch. Hold for 10–15 seconds. Use hands for balance and stability. The farther you move the front foot forward, the more the sole of your foot will rise off the floor.

> A good way to prepare for the splits is to do the stretches on pp. 94–100.

As you become more flexible, continue to move the front foot forward as you lower your hips. Keep your shoulders directly above your hips and your back vertical. Hold for 10–20 seconds. Repeat for the other side.

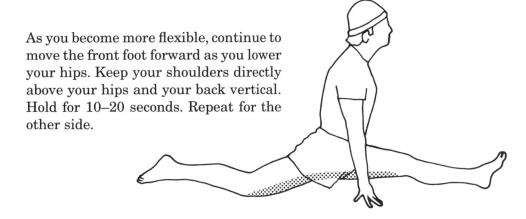

Learning to do the splits takes time and regular practice. Be sure not to overstretch. Let your body gradually adapt to the changes needed to accomplish the splits comfortably. Do not be in a rush and injure yourself.

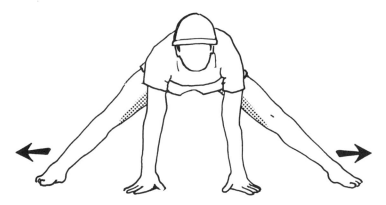

Side Splits

From a standing position, with feet pointed straight ahead, gradually spread your legs until you feel a stretch on the inside of your upper legs. Think of your hips going straight down. Use hands for balance. Hold an easy stretch for at least 15 seconds.

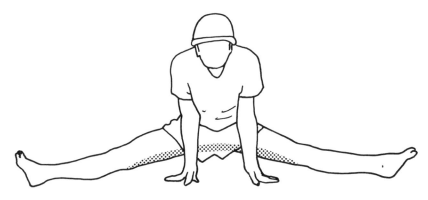

As you become more limber, keep moving your feet apart until the desired stretch is created. As you get lower in this stretch, keep your feet upright, with your heels on the floor: this will keep the stretch on the inside of the upper legs and the extreme tension off the ligaments of the knee. (If you keep your feet flat on the floor there is a possibility of overstretching the inside ligament of the knees.) Hold for 10–20 seconds. As your body gradually adapts, slowly increase the stretch by lowering your hips a bit further. *Be careful of overstretching.*

Doing the stretches below will help you in learning the splits.

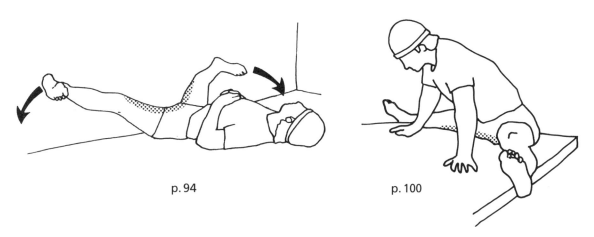

p. 94   p. 100

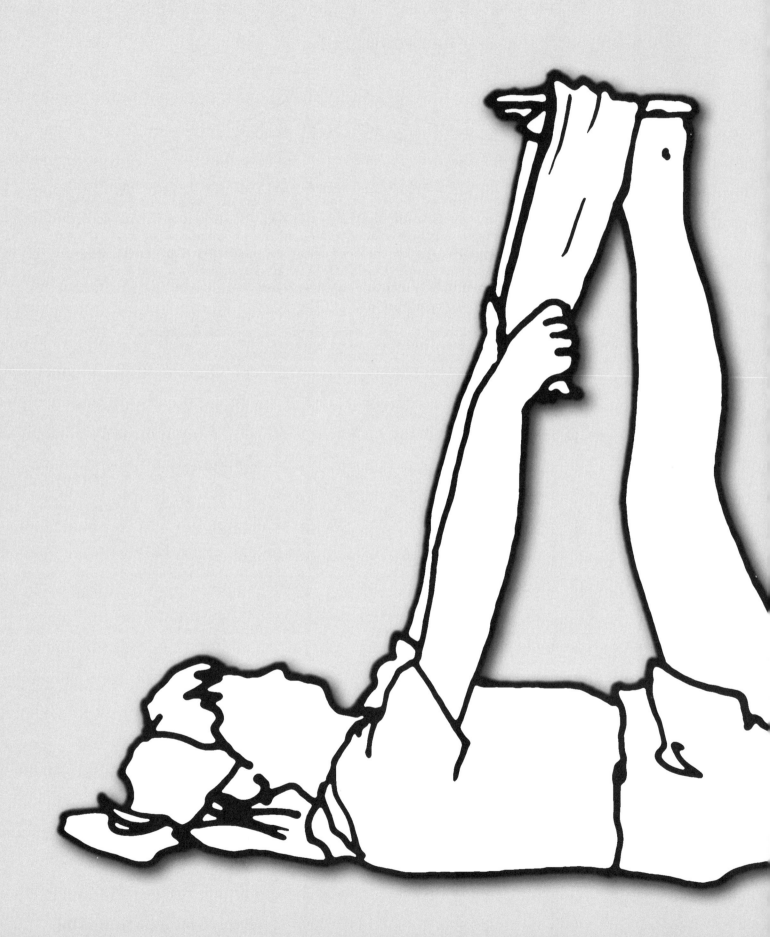

STRETCHING ROUTINES
Everyday Activities

These are stretching routines that can help you in dealing with the muscular tension and tightness of everyday life. There are routines for different age groups, different body parts, different occupations and activities, as well as stretches to do spontaneously at odd moments throughout the day. Once you learn how to stretch, you will be able to develop your own routines to suit your own particular needs.

When you first do the routines, you can look up the instructions for each stretch in the page numbers listed. After a while you will know how to stretch without looking at the instructions each time.

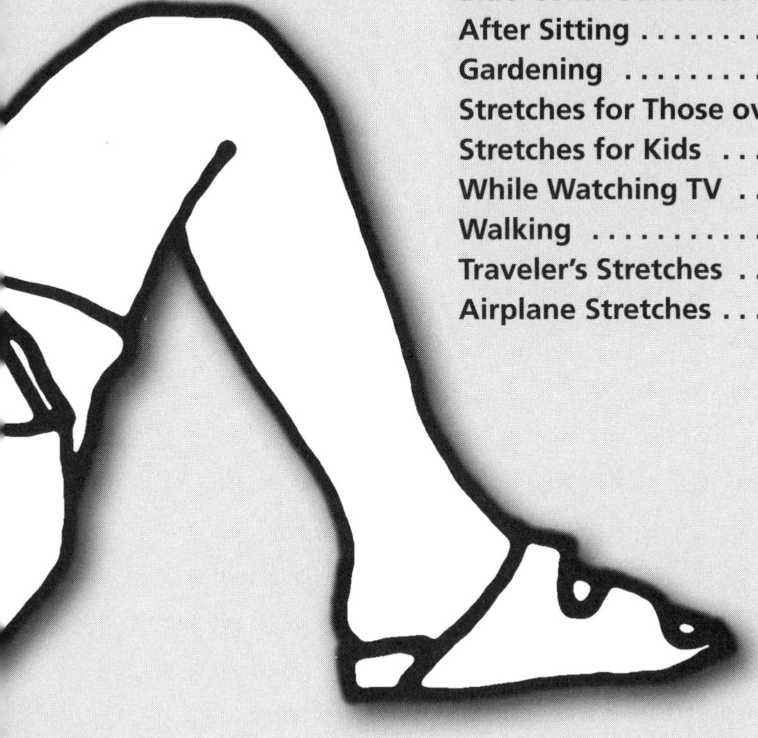

In the Morning

Approximately 4 Minutes

Start the day with some relaxed stretches so your body can function more naturally. Tight and stiff muscles will feel good from comfortable stretching. The first four stretches can be done in bed before you get up. After arising and you've moved around a bit, do the next four stretches.

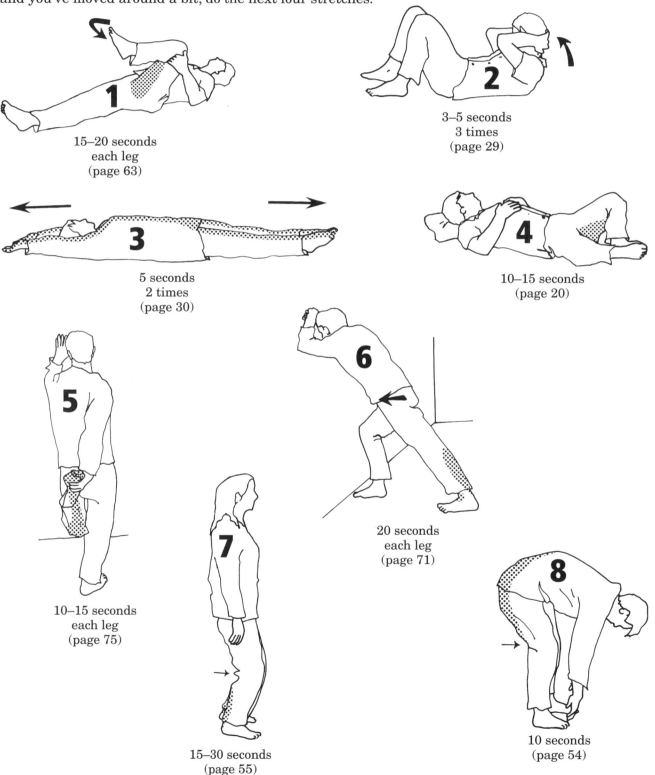

15–20 seconds
each leg
(page 63)

3–5 seconds
3 times
(page 29)

5 seconds
2 times
(page 30)

10–15 seconds
(page 20)

10–15 seconds
each leg
(page 75)

15–30 seconds
(page 55)

20 seconds
each leg
(page 71)

10 seconds
(page 54)

Approximately 3 Minutes

This is a great time to stretch every day. These stretches will relax your
body and help you to sleep more soundly. Take your time, and *feel* the
body parts being stretched. Stretch lightly, breathe deeply, and be relaxed.

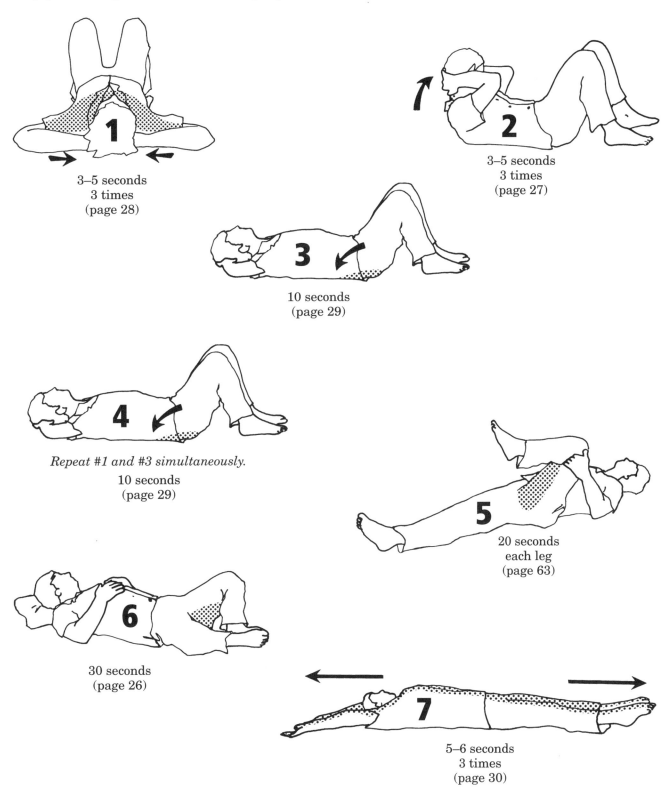

3–5 seconds
3 times
(page 28)

3–5 seconds
3 times
(page 27)

10 seconds
(page 29)

Repeat #1 and #3 simultaneously.
10 seconds
(page 29)

20 seconds
each leg
(page 63)

30 seconds
(page 26)

5–6 seconds
3 times
(page 30)

Everyday Stretches

Approximately 8 Minutes

Start with several minutes of walking. Then use these everyday stretches to fine-tune your muscles. This is a general routine that emphasizes stretching and relaxing the muscles most frequently used during normal day-to-day activities.

In the simple tasks of everyday living, we often use our body in strained or awkward ways, creating stress and tension. A kind of muscular *rigor mortis* sets in. If you can set aside 10 minutes every day for stretching, you will offset this accumulated tension so you can use your body with greater ease.

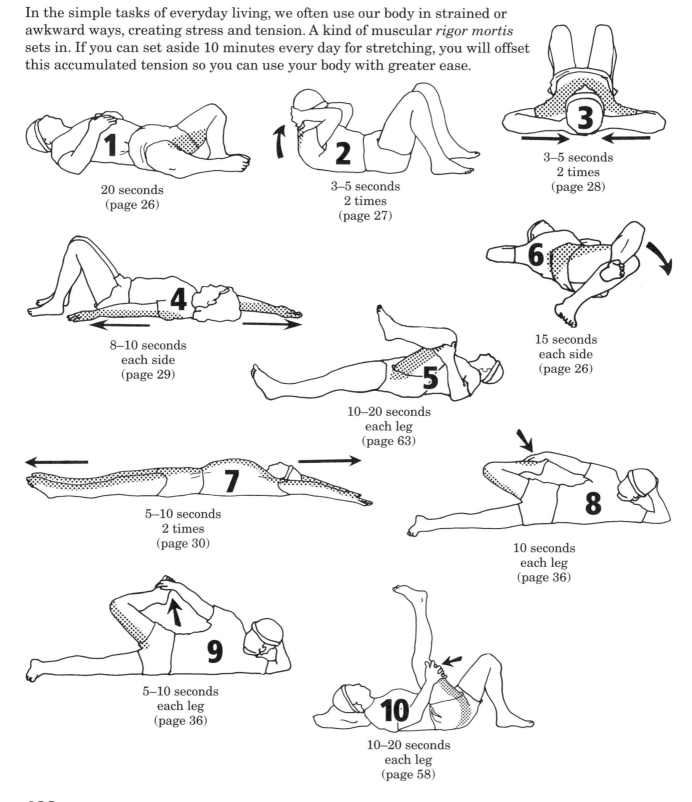

1 — 20 seconds (page 26)

2 — 3–5 seconds 2 times (page 27)

3 — 3–5 seconds 2 times (page 28)

4 — 8–10 seconds each side (page 29)

5 — 10–20 seconds each leg (page 63)

6 — 15 seconds each side (page 26)

7 — 5–10 seconds 2 times (page 30)

8 — 10 seconds each leg (page 36)

9 — 5–10 seconds each leg (page 36)

10 — 10–20 seconds each leg (page 58)

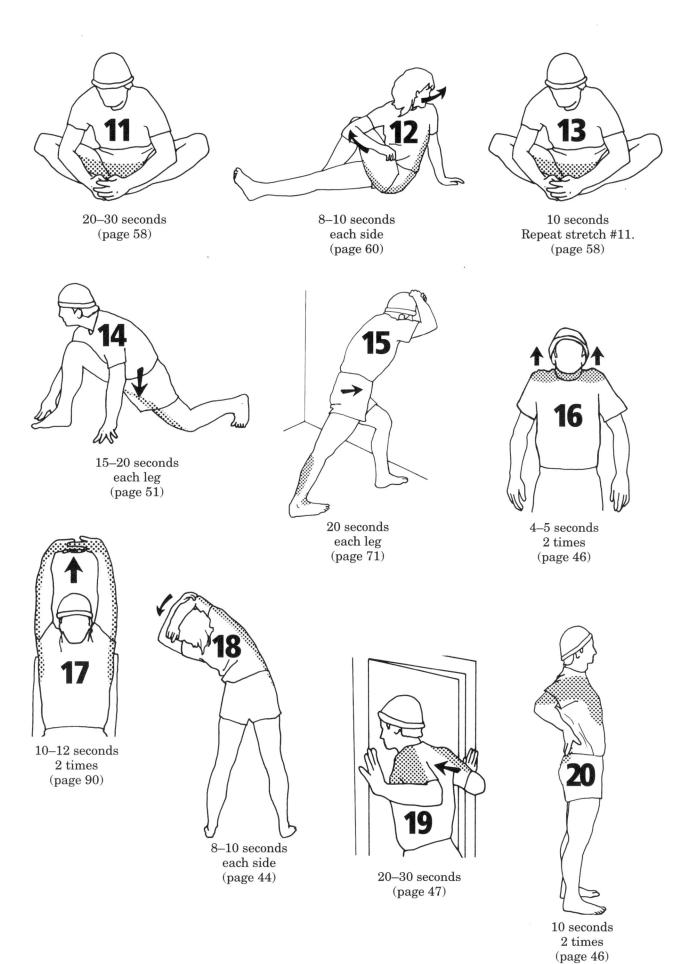

11
20–30 seconds
(page 58)

12
8–10 seconds
each side
(page 60)

13
10 seconds
Repeat stretch #11.
(page 58)

14
15–20 seconds
each leg
(page 51)

15
20 seconds
each leg
(page 71)

16
4–5 seconds
2 times
(page 46)

17
10–12 seconds
2 times
(page 90)

18
8–10 seconds
each side
(page 44)

19
20–30 seconds
(page 47)

20
10 seconds
2 times
(page 46)

Stretches for the
Hands, Arms & Shoulders
Approximately 4 Minutes

This series of stretches works for repetitive stress problems in the hands and arms. Breathe naturally, stay comfortable, and be relaxed as you stretch.

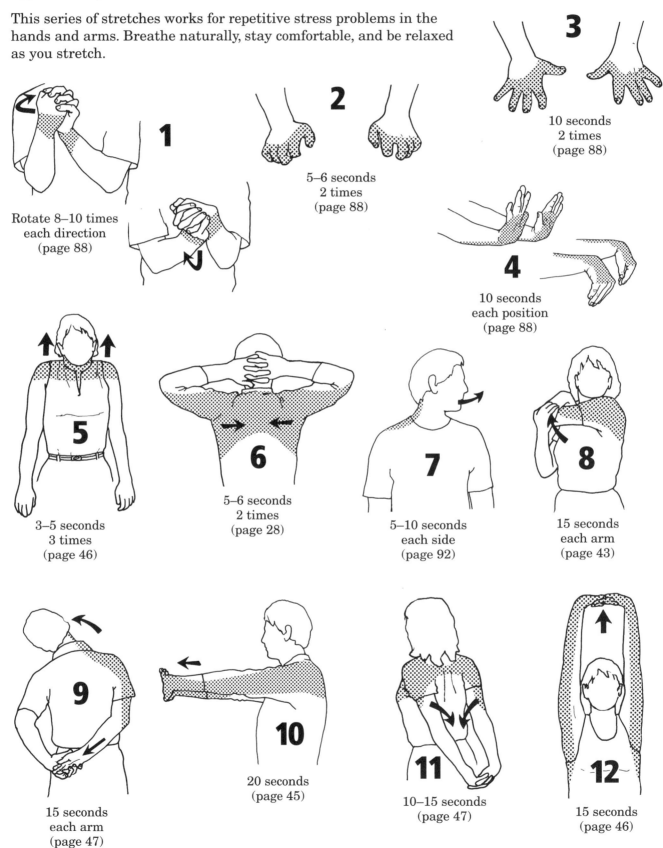

1
Rotate 8–10 times
each direction
(page 88)

2
5–6 seconds
2 times
(page 88)

3
10 seconds
2 times
(page 88)

4
10 seconds
each position
(page 88)

5
3–5 seconds
3 times
(page 46)

6
5–6 seconds
2 times
(page 28)

7
5–10 seconds
each side
(page 92)

8
15 seconds
each arm
(page 43)

9
15 seconds
each arm
(page 47)

10
20 seconds
(page 45)

11
10–15 seconds
(page 47)

12
15 seconds
(page 46)

Stretching © 2000 by Bob and Jean Anderson. Shelter Publications, Inc.

Stretches for the
Neck, Shoulders & Arms
Approximately 5 Minutes

Many people carry stress in their neck and shoulder area. This stretching routine will help with that problem. Do these stretches throughout the day. Breathe deeply and relax.

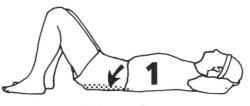

5–6 seconds
(page 29)

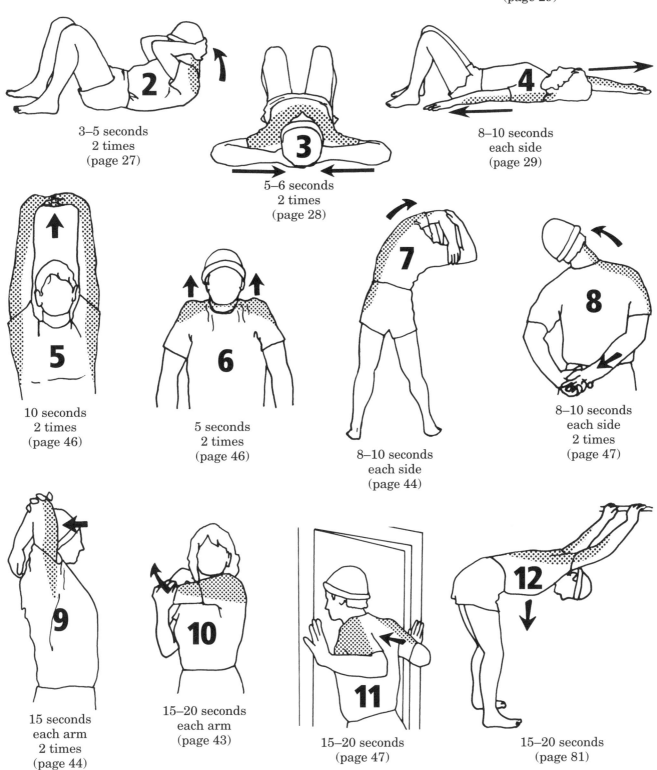

3–5 seconds
2 times
(page 27)

5–6 seconds
2 times
(page 28)

8–10 seconds
each side
(page 29)

10 seconds
2 times
(page 46)

5 seconds
2 times
(page 46)

8–10 seconds
each side
(page 44)

8–10 seconds
each side
2 times
(page 47)

15 seconds
each arm
2 times
(page 44)

15–20 seconds
each arm
(page 43)

15–20 seconds
(page 47)

15–20 seconds
(page 81)

Stretches for the
Legs, Groin & Hips
Approximately 7 Minutes

Stretch comfortably after a light warm-up of walking in place or riding a stationary bike for 2–3 minutes. Remember to stretch with control as you gradually limber up. Relax and breathe rhythmically.

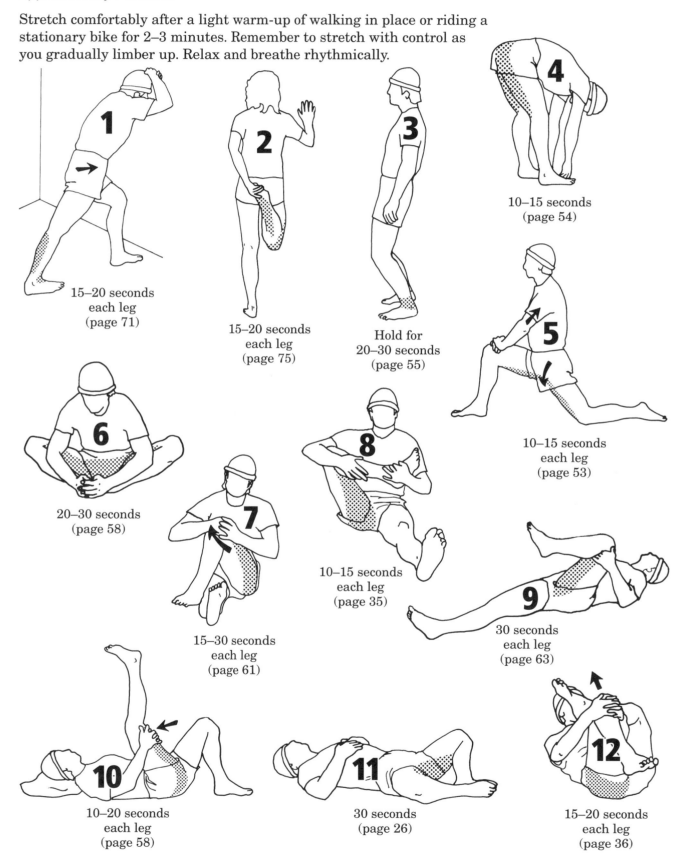

15–20 seconds
each leg
(page 71)

15–20 seconds
each leg
(page 75)

Hold for
20–30 seconds
(page 55)

10–15 seconds
(page 54)

10–15 seconds
each leg
(page 53)

20–30 seconds
(page 58)

15–30 seconds
each leg
(page 61)

10–15 seconds
each leg
(page 35)

30 seconds
each leg
(page 63)

10–20 seconds
each leg
(page 58)

30 seconds
(page 26)

15–20 seconds
each leg
(page 36)

Stretches for
Lower Back Tension
Approximately 6 Minutes

These stretches are designed for the relief of muscular low back pain and are also good for relieving tension in the upper back, shoulders, and neck. For best results do them every night just before going to sleep. Hold only stretch tensions that feel good to you. *Do not overstretch.*

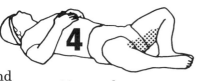

30 seconds
(page 26)

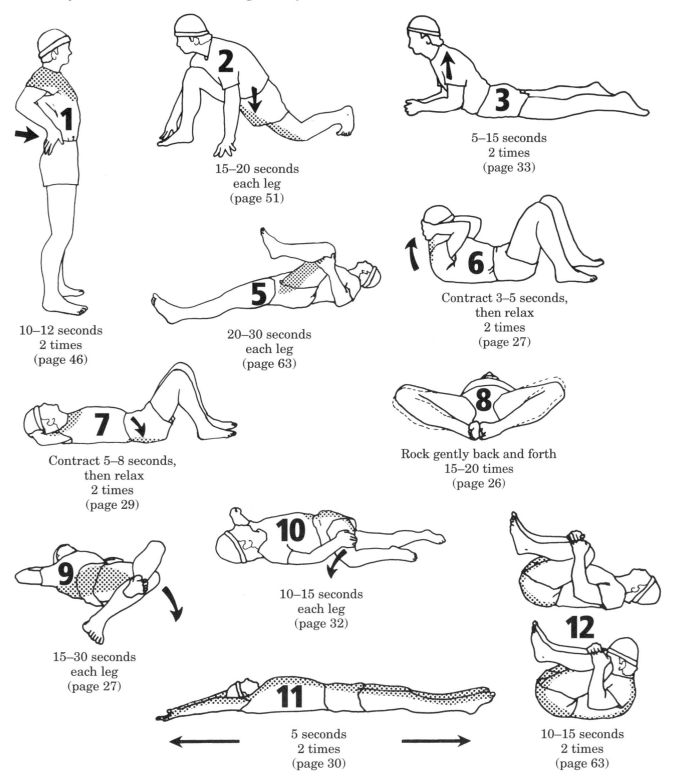

10–12 seconds
2 times
(page 46)

15–20 seconds
each leg
(page 51)

5–15 seconds
2 times
(page 33)

20–30 seconds
each leg
(page 63)

Contract 3–5 seconds,
then relax
2 times
(page 27)

Contract 5–8 seconds,
then relax
2 times
(page 29)

Rock gently back and forth
15–20 times
(page 26)

15–30 seconds
each leg
(page 27)

10–15 seconds
each leg
(page 32)

5 seconds
2 times
(page 30)

10–15 seconds
2 times
(page 63)

Computer & Desk Stretches

Approximately 4 Minutes

Sitting at a computer for long periods often causes neck and shoulder stiffness and occasionally lower back pain. Do these stretches every hour or so throughout the day, or whenever you feel stiff. Photocopy this and keep it in a drawer. Also, be sure to get up and walk around the office whenever you think of it. You'll feel better!

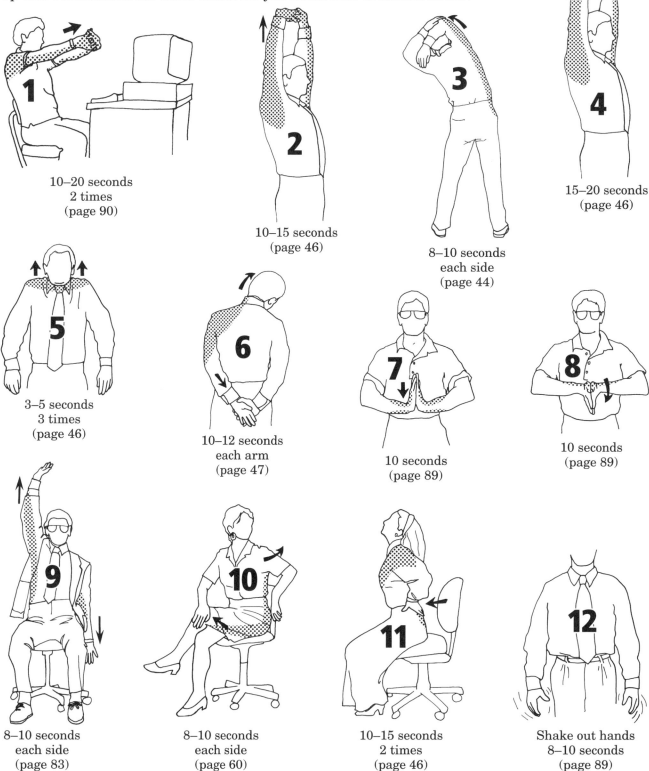

1 — 10–20 seconds
2 times
(page 90)

2 — 10–15 seconds
(page 46)

3 — 8–10 seconds
each side
(page 44)

4 — 15–20 seconds
(page 46)

5 — 3–5 seconds
3 times
(page 46)

6 — 10–12 seconds
each arm
(page 47)

7 — 10 seconds
(page 89)

8 — 10 seconds
(page 89)

9 — 8–10 seconds
each side
(page 83)

10 — 8–10 seconds
each side
(page 60)

11 — 10–15 seconds
2 times
(page 46)

12 — Shake out hands
8–10 seconds
(page 89)

Stretching © 2000 by Bob and Jean Anderson. Shelter Publications, Inc.

Spontaneous Stretches

You can stretch at odd times of the day. Reading a paper, talking on the phone, waiting for a bus . . . these are times for easy, relaxed stretching. Be creative; think of stretches to do during normally wasted time.

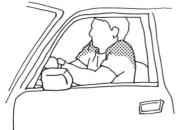

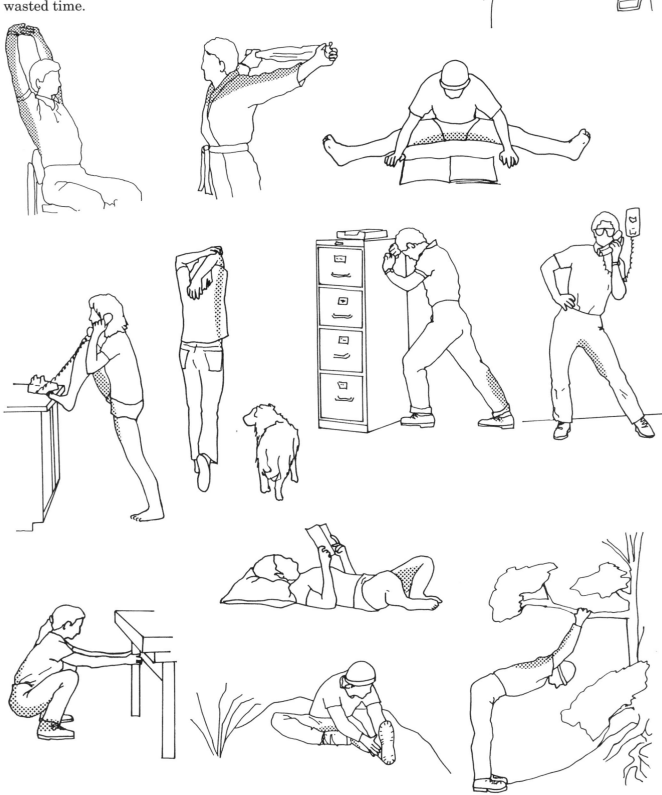

Blue-Collar Stretches

Approximately 6 Minutes

Before you do any physical work—especially lifting—do some stretches. Stretching gives your muscles a signal they are about to be used, and a few minutes of stretching before starting work will make you feel better and help avoid injuries.

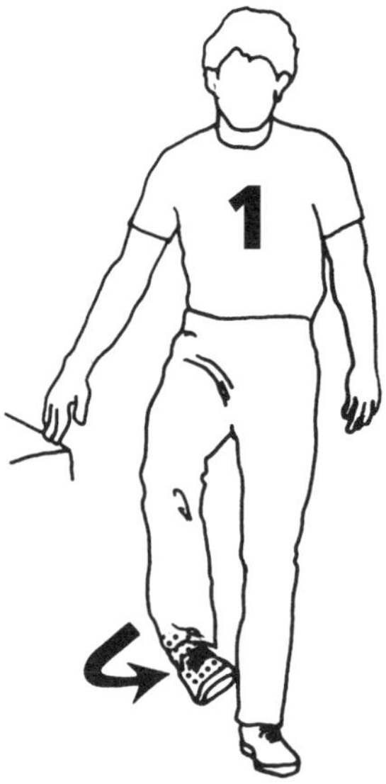

1

10–20 times
each foot
(page 71)

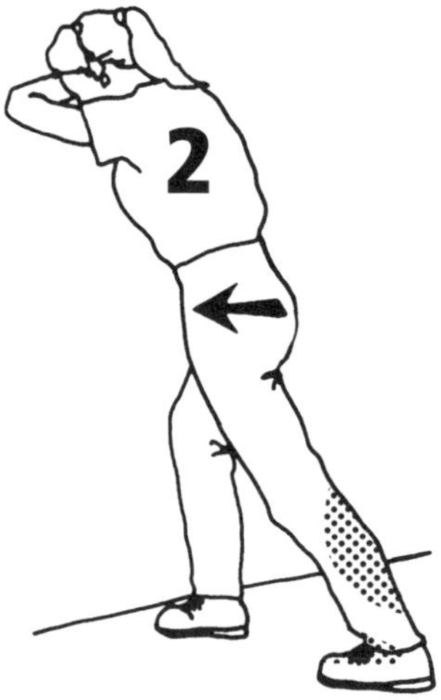

2

10–20 seconds
each leg
(page 71)

3

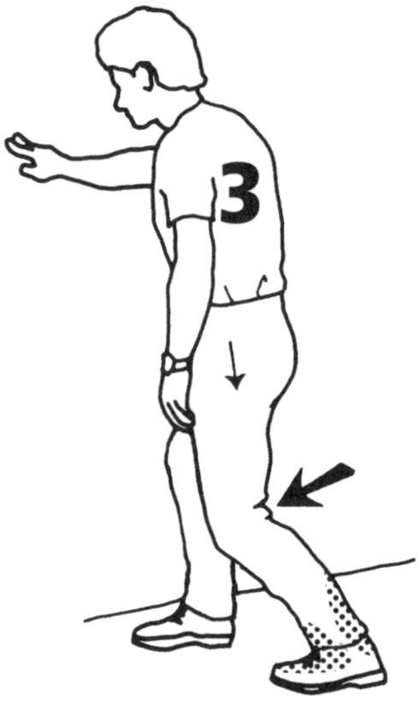

5–10 seconds
each leg
(page 71)

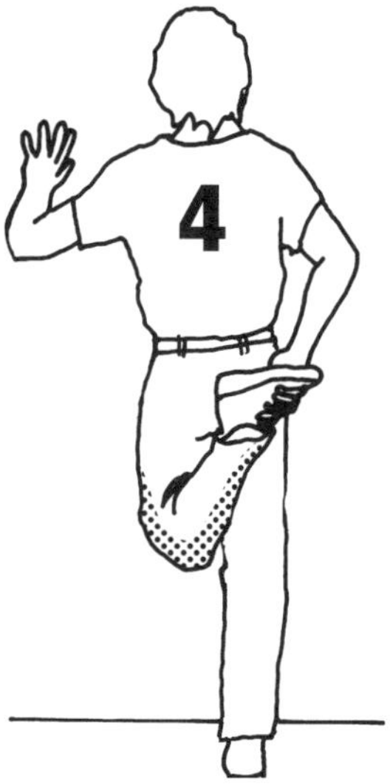

4

10 seconds
each leg
(page 75)

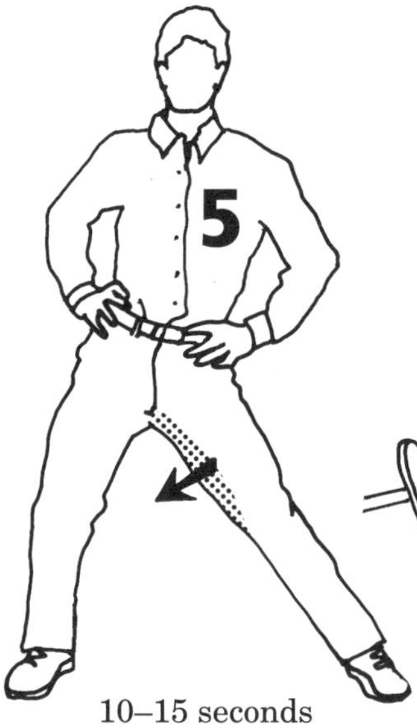

5

10–15 seconds
each leg
(page 73)

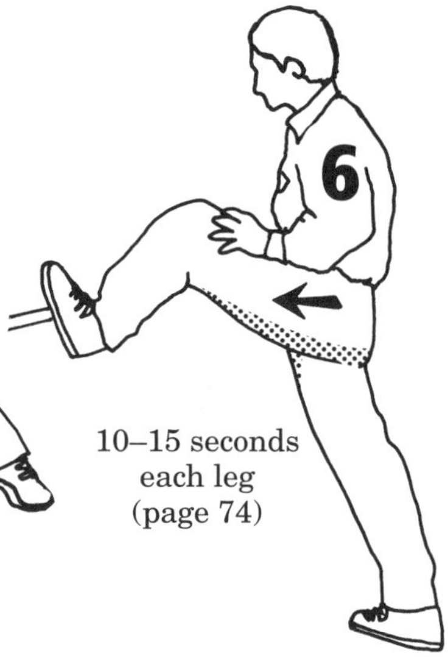

6

10–15 seconds
each leg
(page 74)

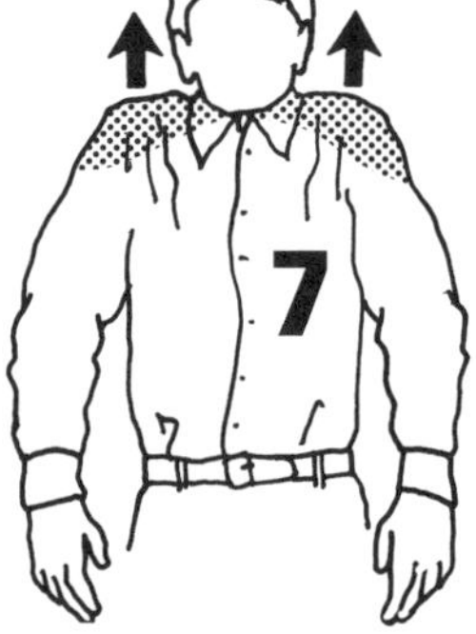

7

3–5 seconds
2 times
(page 46)

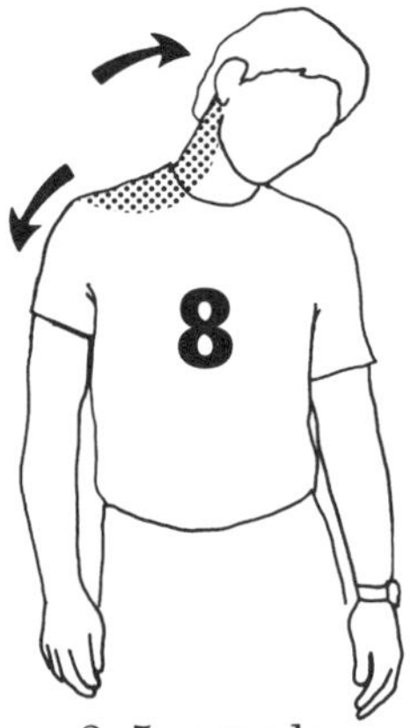

8

3–5 seconds
each side
(page 46)

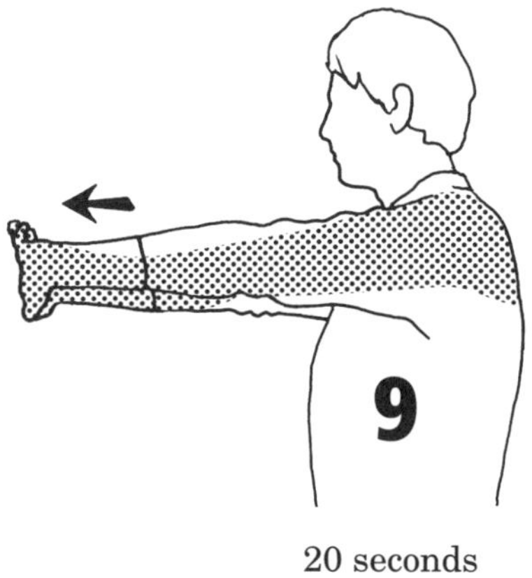

9

20 seconds
(page 45)

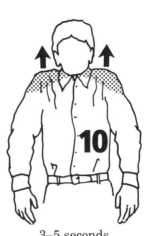

3–5 seconds
(page 46)

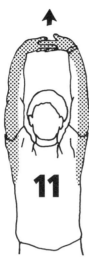

10 seconds
(page 46)

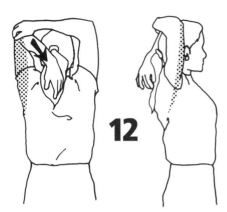

10 seconds
each arm
(page 44)

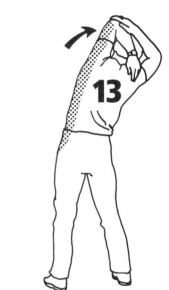

8–10 seconds
each side
(page 44)

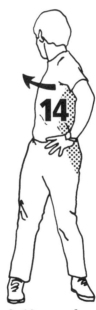

8–10 seconds
each side
(page 81)

8–10 seconds
2 times
(page 46)

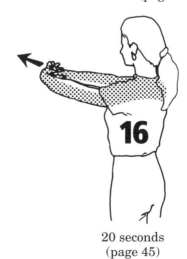

20 seconds
(page 45)

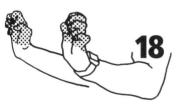

8–10 seconds
2 times
(page 88)

5–8 seconds
2 times
(page 88)

After
Sitting
Approximately 4 Minutes

This is a series of stretches to do after sitting for a long time. The sitting position causes the blood to pool in the lower legs and feet, the hamstring muscles to tighten up, and the back and neck muscles to become stiff and tight. These stretches will improve your circulation and loosen up those areas that are tense from a prolonged period of sitting.

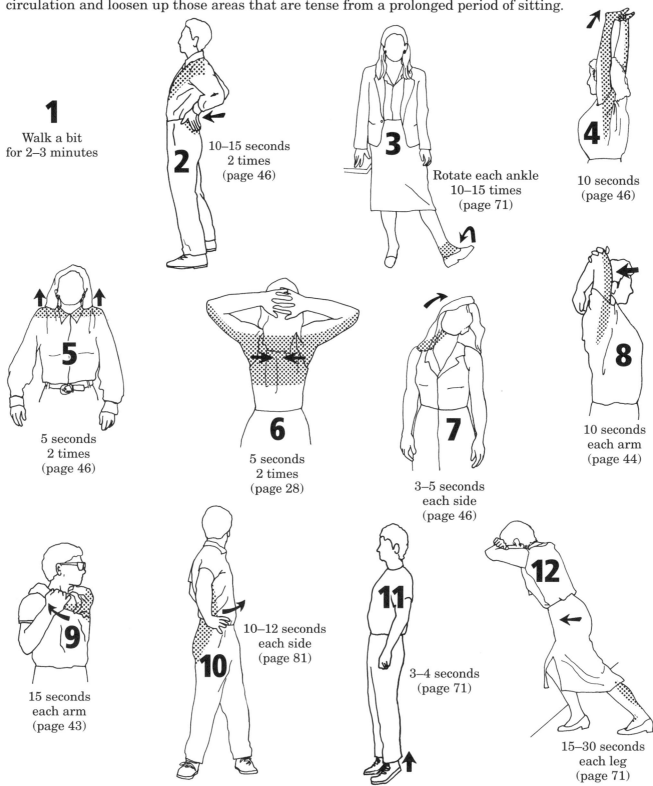

1
Walk a bit
for 2–3 minutes

2
10–15 seconds
2 times
(page 46)

3
Rotate each ankle
10–15 times
(page 71)

4
10 seconds
(page 46)

5
5 seconds
2 times
(page 46)

6
5 seconds
2 times
(page 28)

7
3–5 seconds
each side
(page 46)

8
10 seconds
each arm
(page 44)

9
15 seconds
each arm
(page 43)

10
10–12 seconds
each side
(page 81)

11
3–4 seconds
(page 71)

12
15–30 seconds
each leg
(page 71)

Before and After
Gardening
Approximately 4 Minutes

Before you do any work in the garden, do a few minutes of easy stretching. This will help get your body ready to work efficiently without the usual tightness and stiffness that results from this kind of work. Stretch to reduce muscle tension and make work easier.

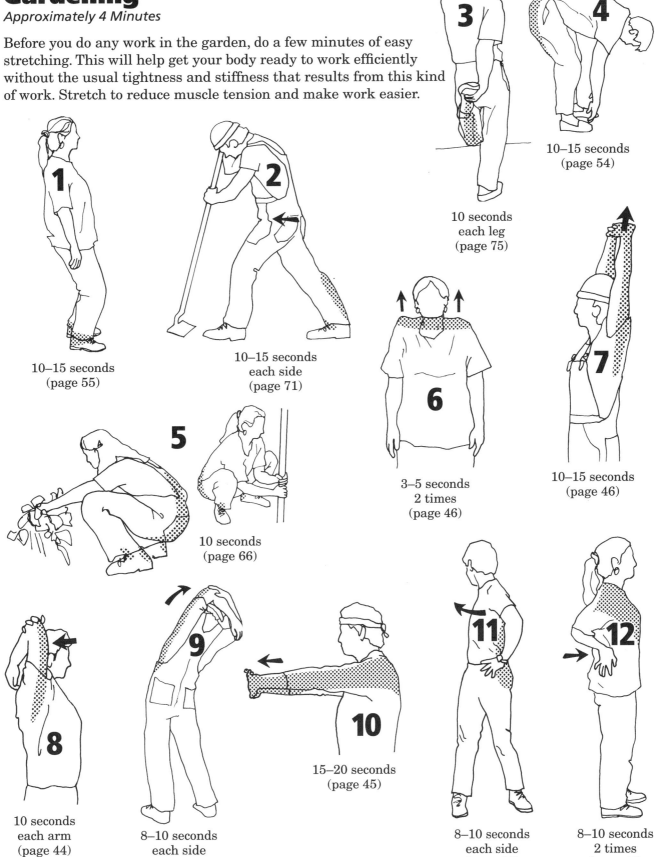

1 10–15 seconds
(page 55)

2 10–15 seconds
each side
(page 71)

3 10 seconds
each leg
(page 75)

4 10–15 seconds
(page 54)

5 10 seconds
(page 66)

6 3–5 seconds
2 times
(page 46)

7 10–15 seconds
(page 46)

8 10 seconds
each arm
(page 44)

9 8–10 seconds
each side
(page 44)

10 15–20 seconds
(page 45)

11 8–10 seconds
each side
(page 81)

12 8–10 seconds
2 times
(page 46)

Stretches for Those
Over 60
Approximately 7 Minutes

It is never too late to start stretching. In fact, the older we get, the more important it becomes to stretch on a regular basis.

With age and inactivity, the body gradually loses its range of motion; muscles can lose their elasticity and become weak and tight. But the body has an amazing capacity for the recovery of lost flexibility and strength if a regular program of fitness is followed.

The basic method of stretching is the same regardless of differences in age and flexibility. *Stretching properly means that you do not go beyond your comfortable limits.* You don't have to try to copy the drawings in this book. Learn to stretch your body without pushing too far; stretch by how you feel. It will take time to loosen up tight muscle groups that have been that way for years, but it can be done with patience and regularity. If you have any doubts about what you should be doing, consult your physician *before you start.*

Here is a series of stretches to help restore and maintain flexibility.

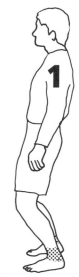

10–30 seconds
(page 55)

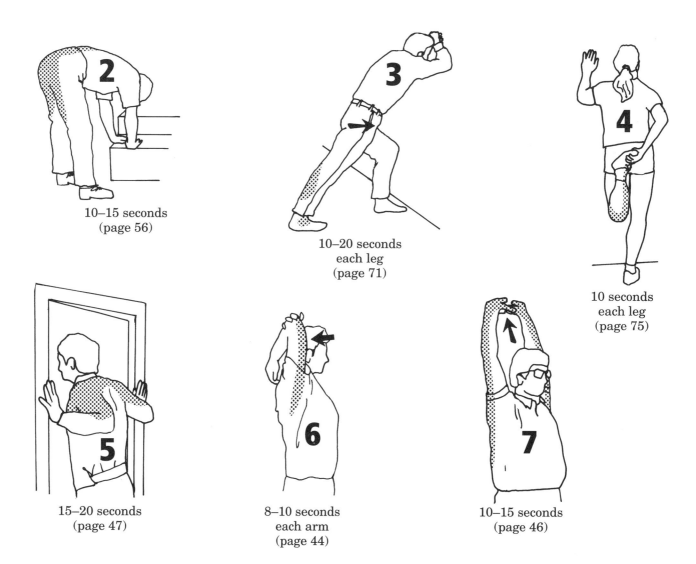

10–15 seconds
(page 56)

10–20 seconds
each leg
(page 71)

10 seconds
each leg
(page 75)

15–20 seconds
(page 47)

8–10 seconds
each arm
(page 44)

10–15 seconds
(page 46)

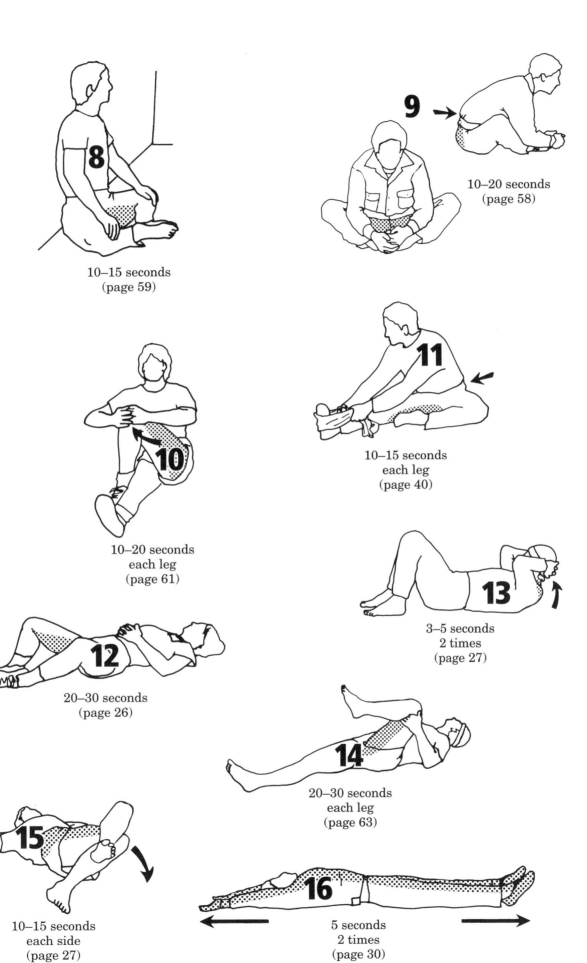

8

10–15 seconds
(page 59)

9

10–20 seconds
(page 58)

10

10–20 seconds
each leg
(page 61)

11

10–15 seconds
each leg
(page 40)

12

20–30 seconds
(page 26)

13

3–5 seconds
2 times
(page 27)

14

20–30 seconds
each leg
(page 63)

15

10–15 seconds
each side
(page 27)

16

5 seconds
2 times
(page 30)

Stretches for
Kids
Approximately 5 Minutes

It's never too early to start stretching! Show your kids how to do these stretches (or show these to your kids' teachers, so they can get the whole class stretching). Explain to them that stretching is not a contest, and that they should stretch slowly, concentrating on the areas being stretched.

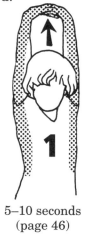

5–10 seconds
(page 46)

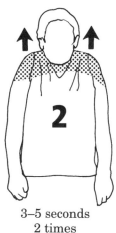

3–5 seconds
2 times
(page 46)

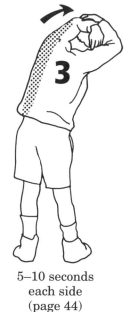

5–10 seconds
each side
(page 44)

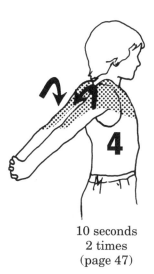

10 seconds
2 times
(page 47)

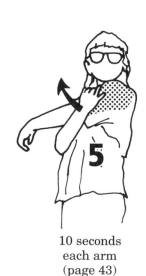

10 seconds
each arm
(page 43)

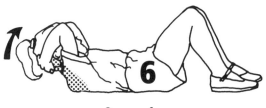

3 seconds
2 times
(page 27)

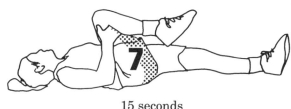

15 seconds
each leg
(page 63)

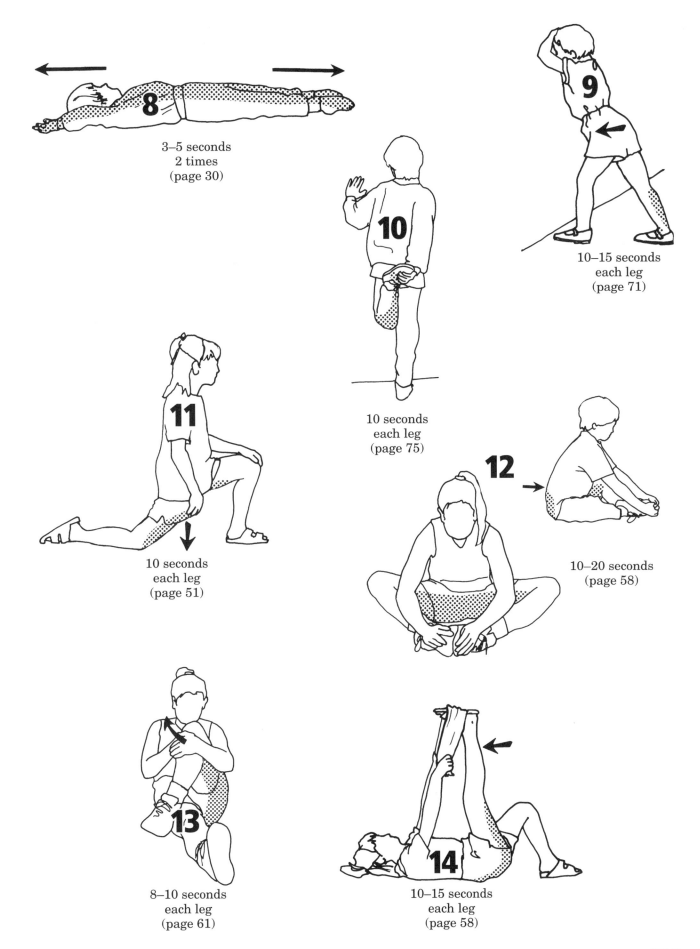

8

3–5 seconds
2 times
(page 30)

9

10–15 seconds
each leg
(page 71)

10

10 seconds
each leg
(page 75)

11

10 seconds
each leg
(page 51)

12

10–20 seconds
(page 58)

13

8–10 seconds
each leg
(page 61)

14

10–15 seconds
each leg
(page 58)

While Watching TV

Many people think they don't have enough time to stretch, yet watch several hours of television a night. Well, you can stretch as you watch TV. This will not interfere with your viewing and you will be accomplishing something during otherwise sedentary times.

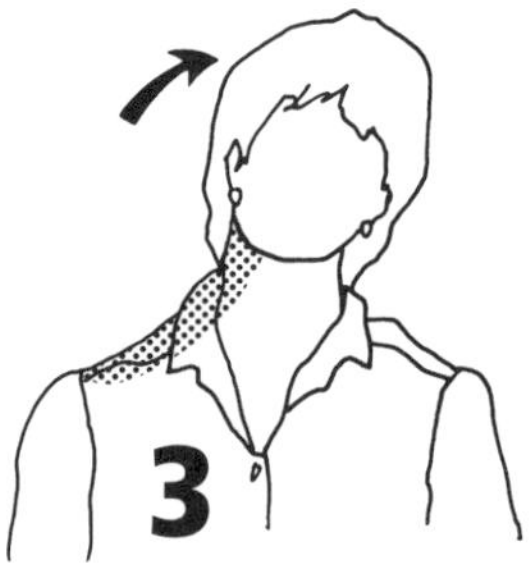

3

3–5 seconds
each side
(page 46)

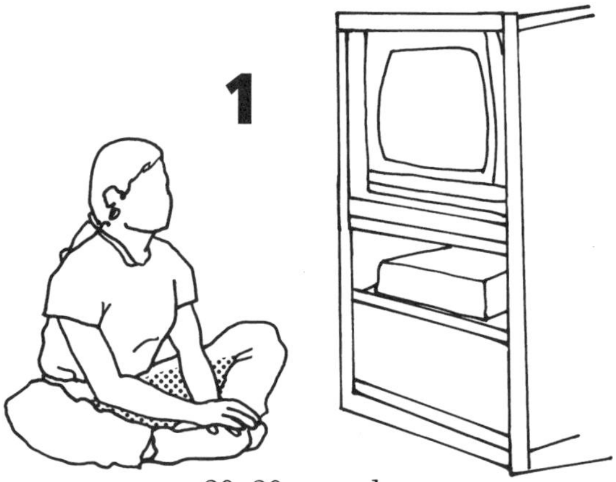

1

20–30 seconds
(page 58)

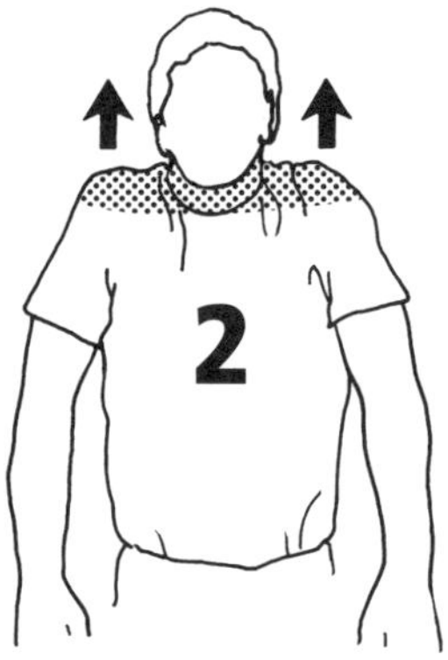

2

3–5 seconds
3 times
(page 46)

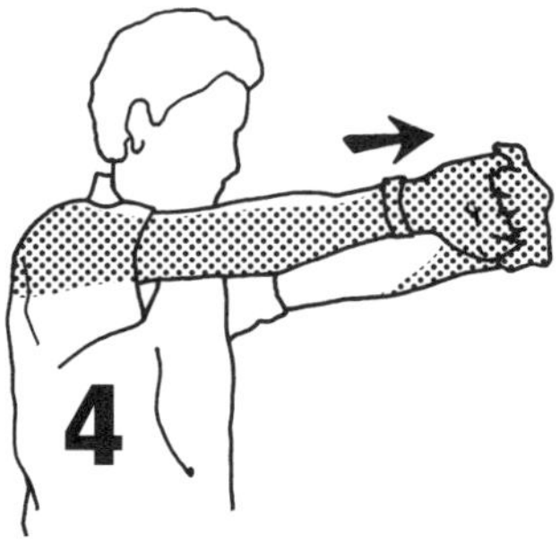

4

15 seconds
(page 45)

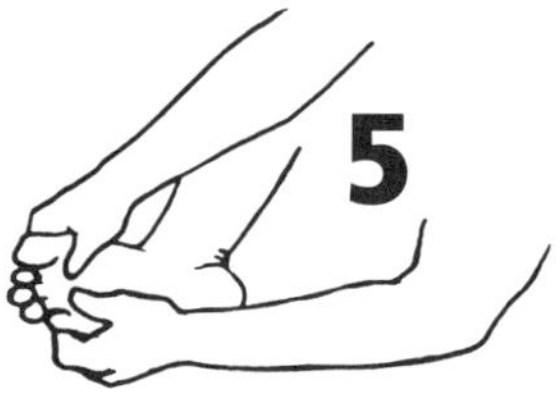

5

30–60 seconds
each foot
(page 34)

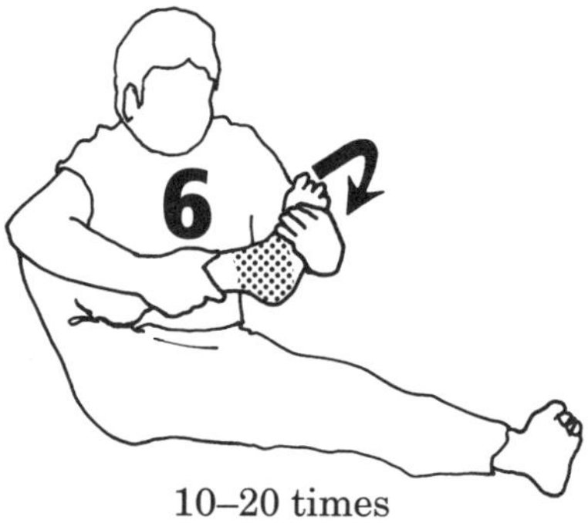

6

10–20 times
each foot
(page 34)

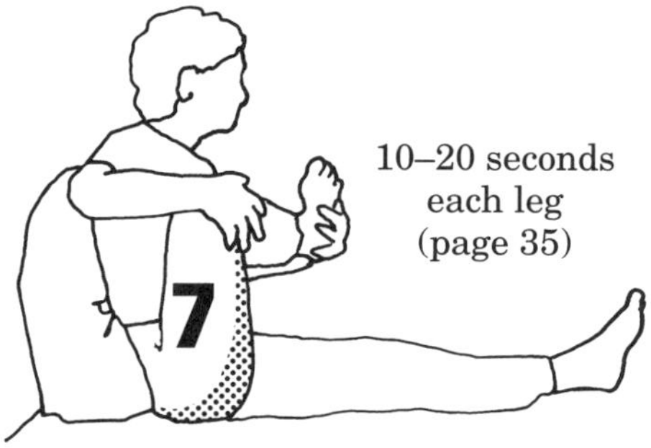

7

10–20 seconds
each leg
(page 35)

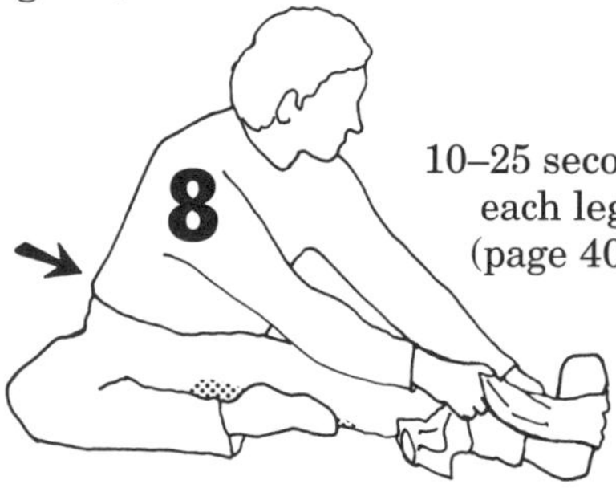

8

10–25 seconds
each leg
(page 40)

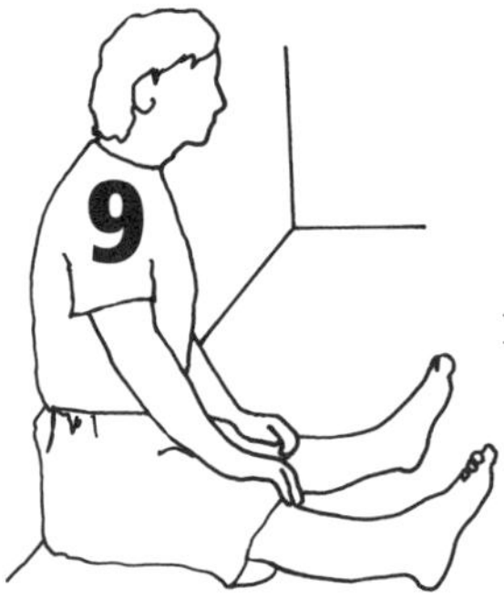

9

10–30 seconds
(page 98)

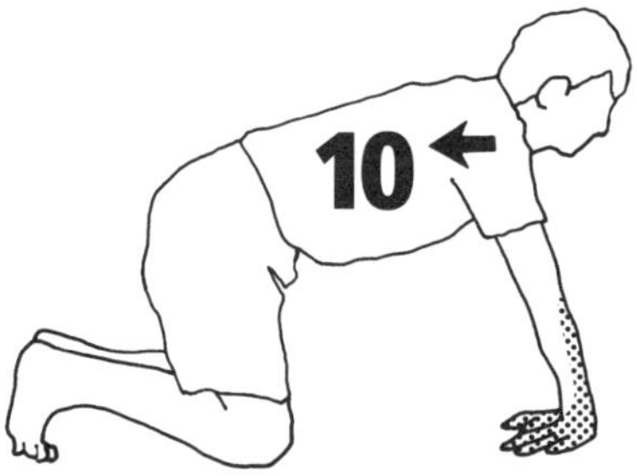

10

10–20 seconds
(page 42)

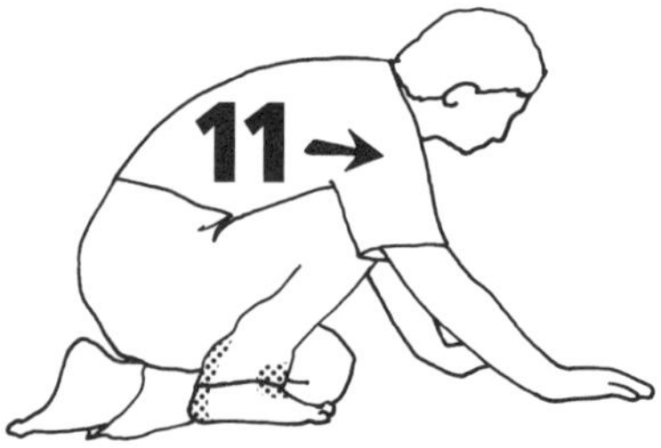

11

5–10 seconds
each leg
(page 50)

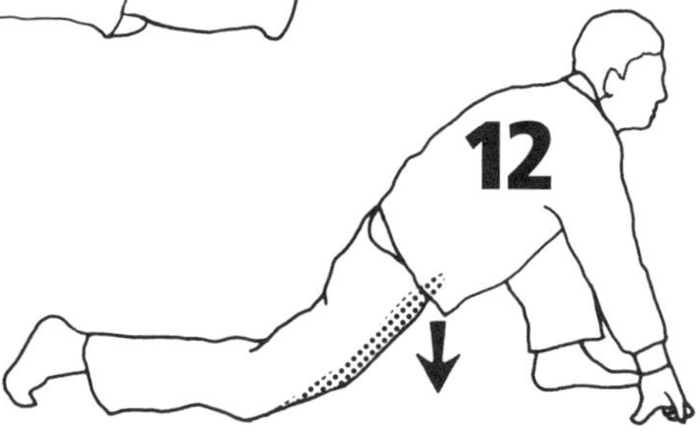

12

10–20 seconds
each leg
(page 51)

Before and After
Walking
Approximately 5 Minutes

These stretches will make the movements of walking feel free
and easy. Warm up by walking several minutes before stretching.

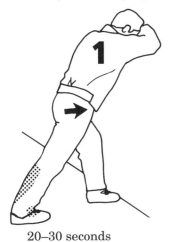

1

20–30 seconds
each leg
(page 71)

2

5–10 seconds
each leg
(page 71)

3

10–15 seconds
each leg
(page 75)

4

20–30 seconds
(page 55)

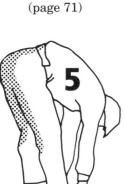

5

10–15 seconds
(page 54)

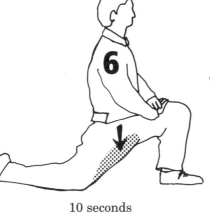

6

10 seconds
each leg
(page 53)

7

10–15 seconds
(page 58)

8

15–20 seconds
each side
(page 61)

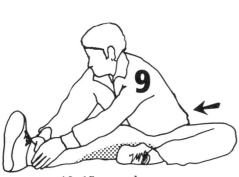

9

10–15 seconds
each leg
(page 39)

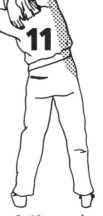

10

10–20 seconds
(page 47)

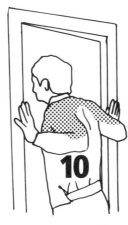

11

8–10 seconds
each side
(page 44)

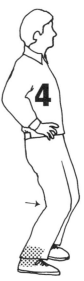
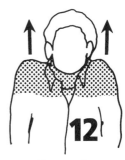
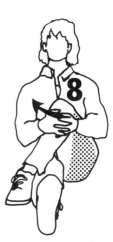

12

5 seconds
2 times
(page 46)

Traveler's Stretches

Approximately 2 Minutes

Stretch at various times throughout your journey to help your body feel less stiff and tight.

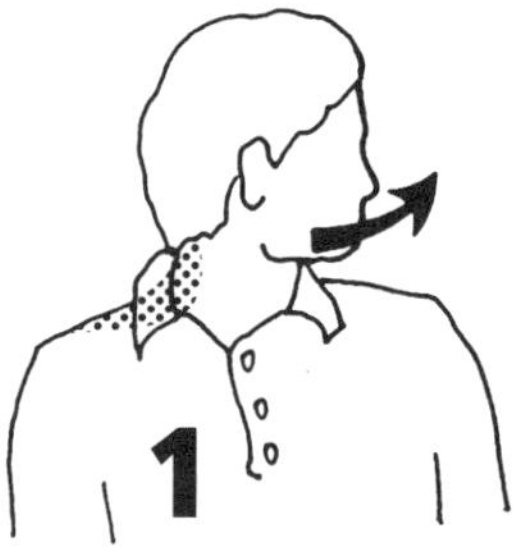

1 3–5 seconds each side (page 92)

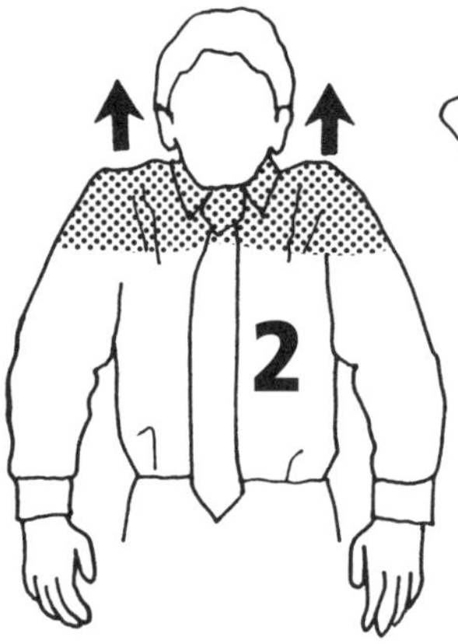

2 3–5 seconds 3 times (page 46)

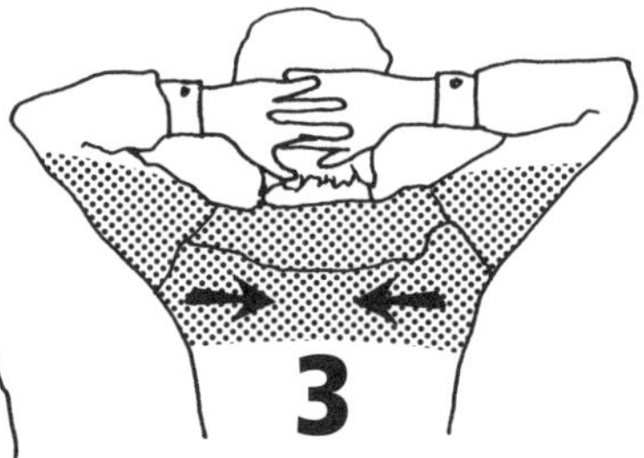

3 3–5 seconds (page 91)

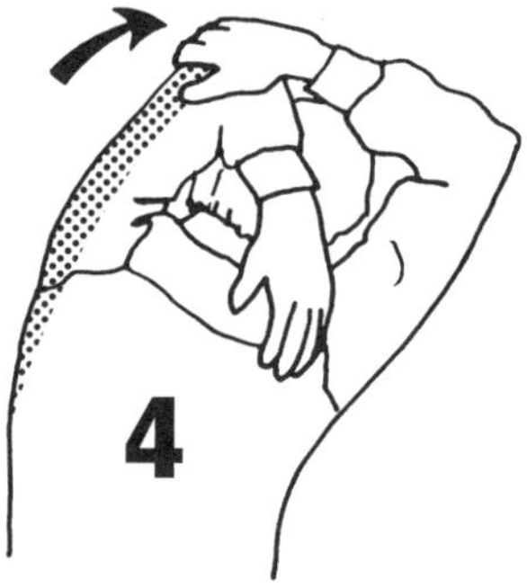

4 5 seconds each side (page 44)

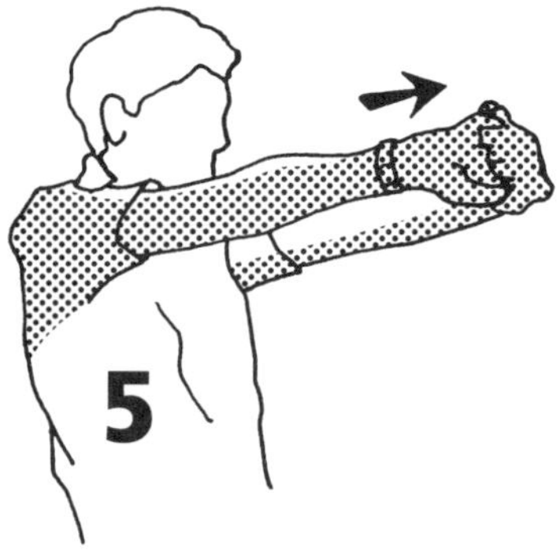

5 15 seconds (page 90)

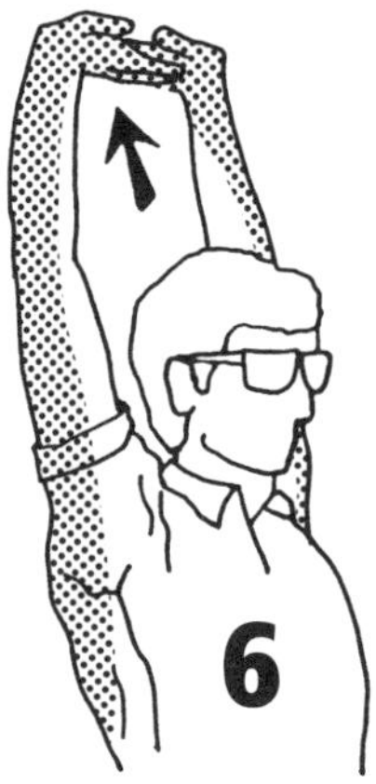

6 8–10 seconds (page 90)

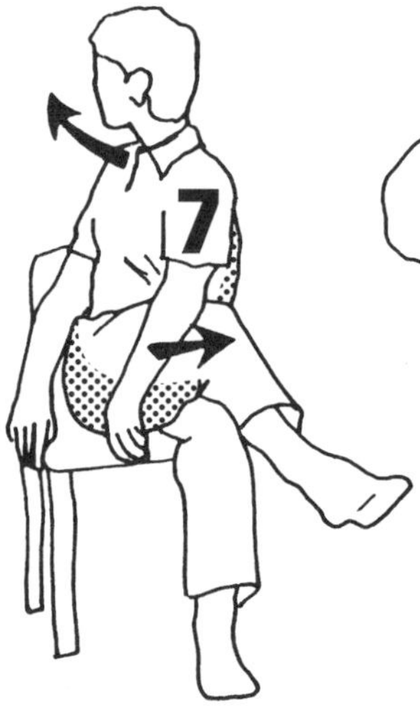

7 8–10 seconds each side (page 60)

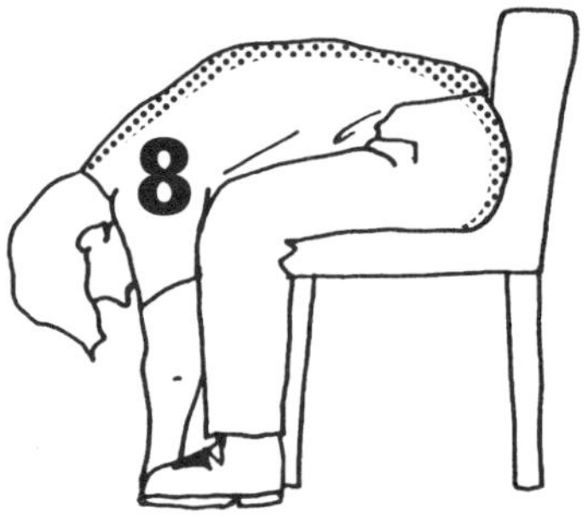

8 5 seconds (page 92)

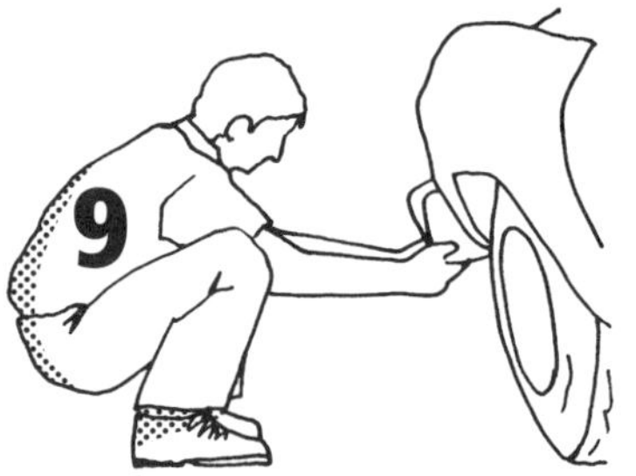

9 10 seconds (page 66)

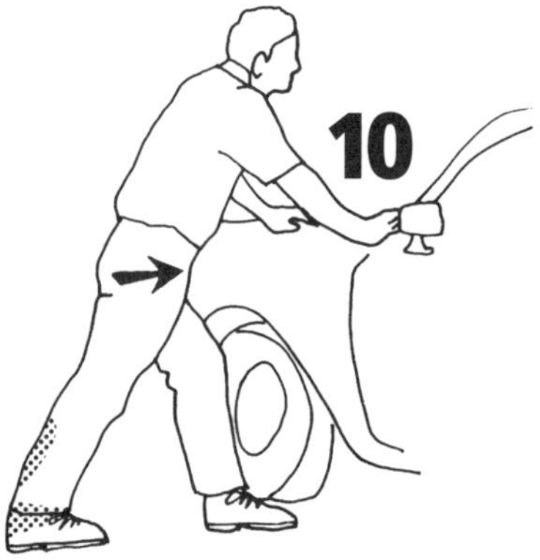

10 10 seconds each leg (page 71)

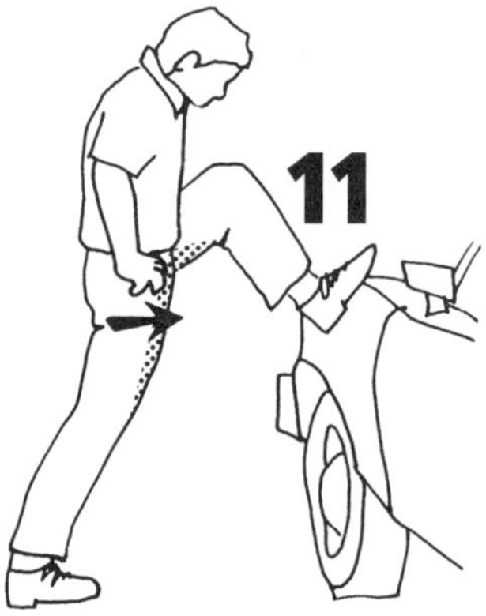

11 8 seconds each leg (page 74)

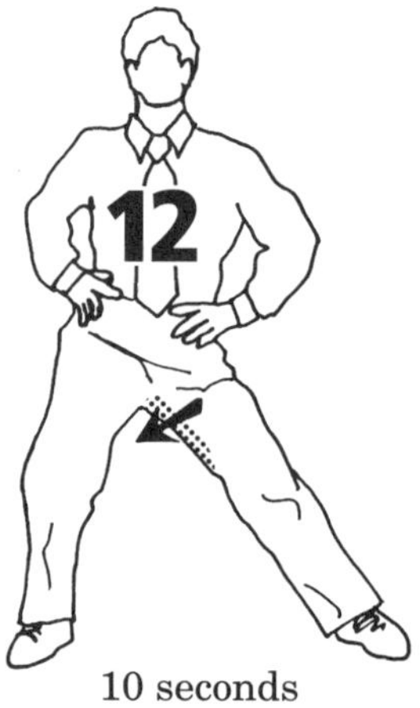

12 10 seconds each leg (page 73)

Stretching © 2000 by Bob and Jean Anderson. Shelter Publications, Inc.

Airplane Stretches

Photocopy this page and take it along on your next flight. Stretching on the plane will relieve stress and stiffness and allow you to arrive in a more relaxed state. Don't be surprised if your fellow passengers follow your example and start stretching too. Especially good to do just before you land.

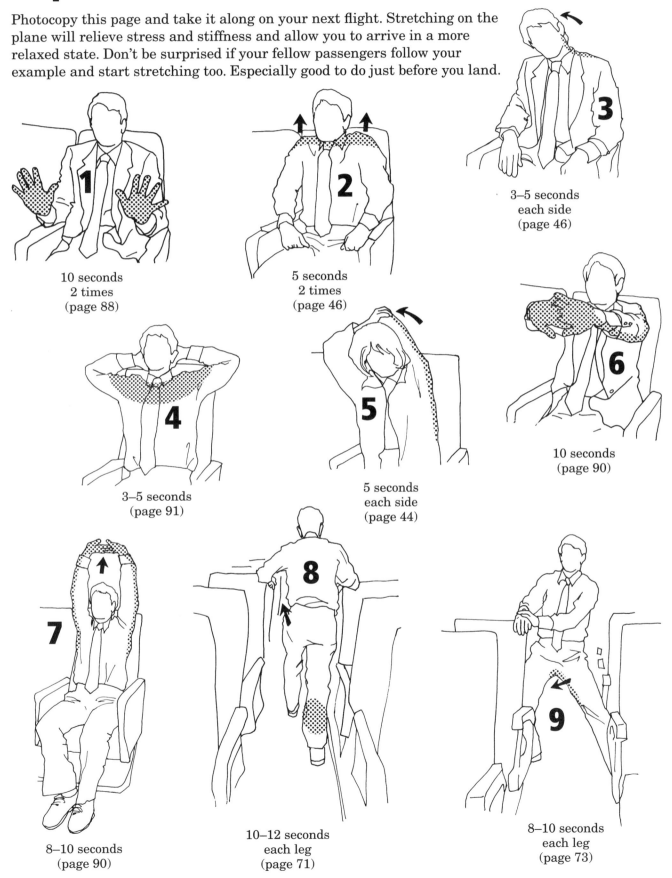

3–5 seconds
each side
(page 46)

10 seconds
2 times
(page 88)

5 seconds
2 times
(page 46)

3–5 seconds
(page 91)

5 seconds
each side
(page 44)

10 seconds
(page 90)

8–10 seconds
(page 90)

10–12 seconds
each leg
(page 71)

8–10 seconds
each leg
(page 73)

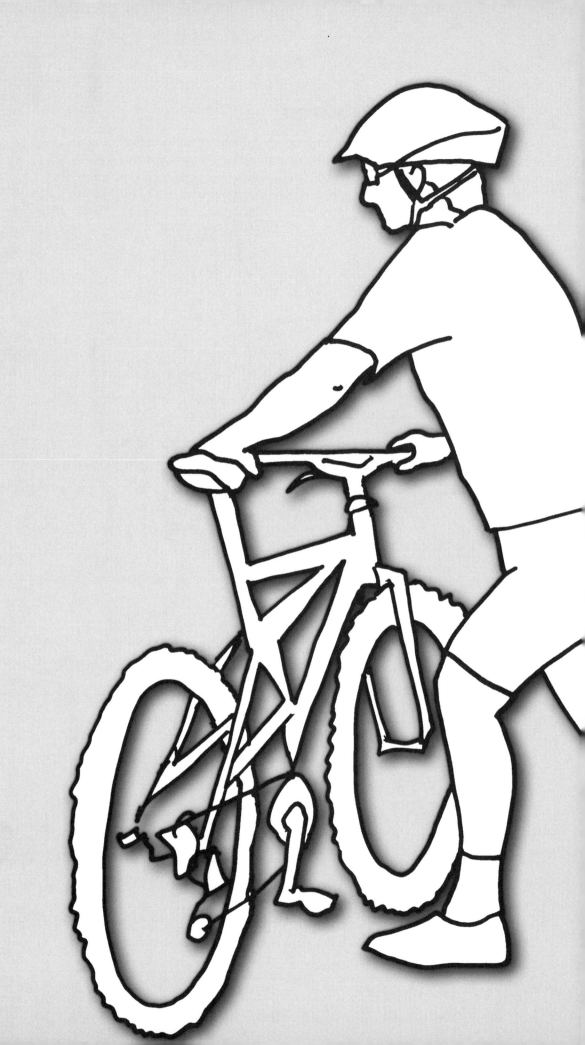

STRETCHING ROUTINES
Sports and Activities

In this section are stretching routines for sports and activities, arranged in alphabetical order.

Each time you do a stretch for the first time, read the *specific* instructions for that stretch. (See the page reference under each stretch.) After you follow the instructions a few times, you'll know how to do each stretch correctly. From then on, simply look at the drawings.

Warming up: For the more vigorous sports (running, football, etc.), I recommend that you do a short warm-up before stretching (jogging for 3–5 minutes with an exaggerated arm swing, for example). See p. 14, Warming Up and Cooling Down.

To teachers and coaches: These routines can serve as guidelines. You can add or subtract stretches to meet specific needs and time allotments.

Note: Be sure to read How To Stretch on pp. 12–13 before you do these routines.

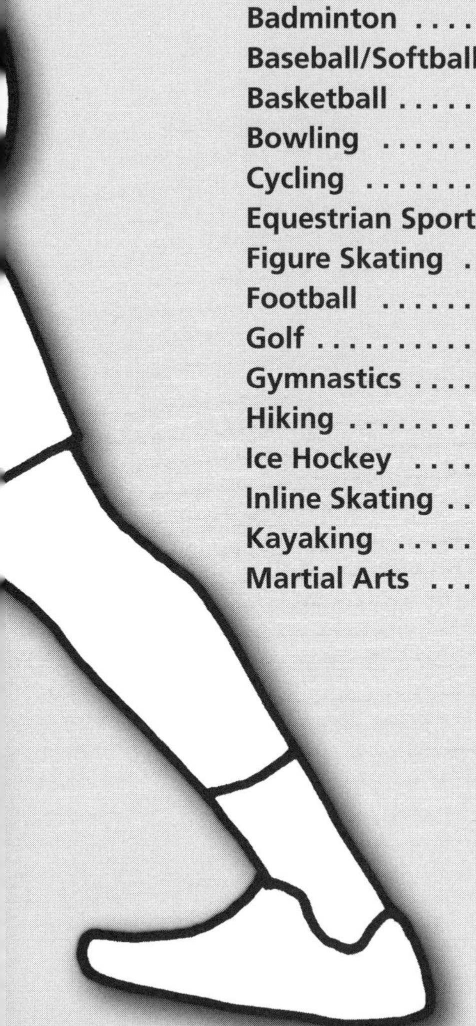

Before and After
Aerobic Exercise
Approximately 6 Minutes

Do a mild warm-up of 2–3 minutes before stretching.

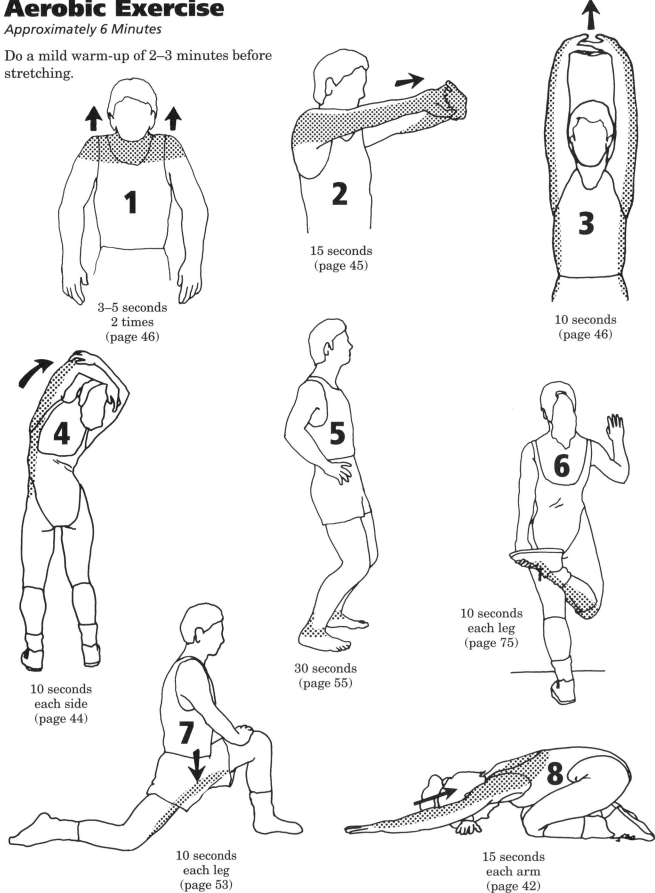

1 3–5 seconds
2 times
(page 46)

2 15 seconds
(page 45)

3 10 seconds
(page 46)

4 10 seconds
each side
(page 44)

5 30 seconds
(page 55)

6 10 seconds
each leg
(page 75)

7 10 seconds
each leg
(page 53)

8 15 seconds
each arm
(page 42)

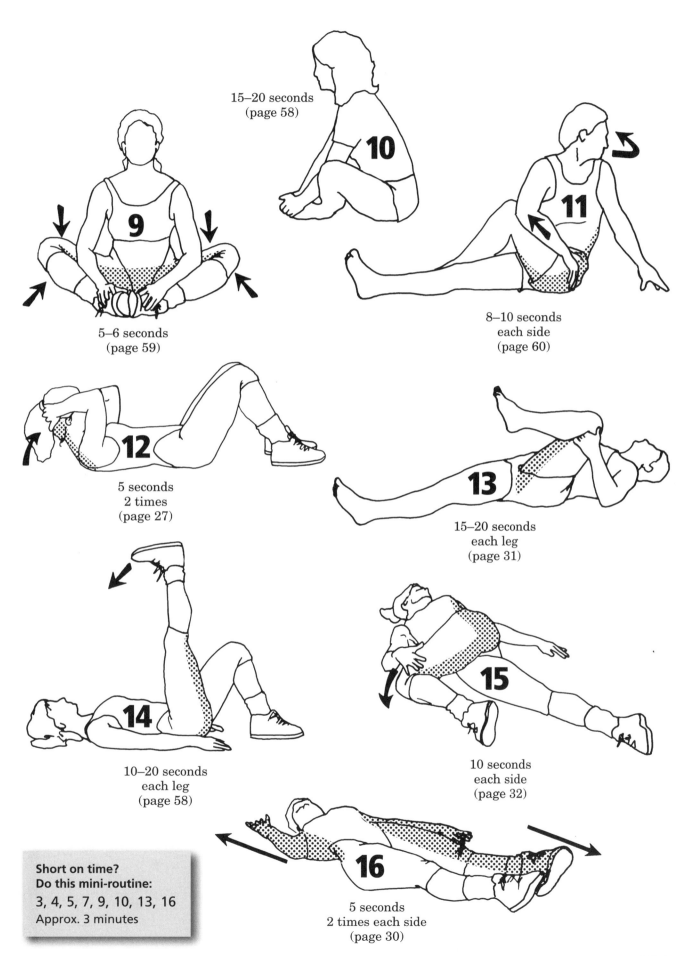

15–20 seconds
(page 58)

10

11

8–10 seconds
each side
(page 60)

9

5–6 seconds
(page 59)

12

5 seconds
2 times
(page 27)

13

15–20 seconds
each leg
(page 31)

14

10–20 seconds
each leg
(page 58)

15

10 seconds
each side
(page 32)

16

5 seconds
2 times each side
(page 30)

Short on time?
Do this mini-routine:
3, 4, 5, 7, 9, 10, 13, 16
Approx. 3 minutes

Before and After
Badminton
Approximately 6 Minutes

Warm up with 2–3 minutes of walking before stretching.

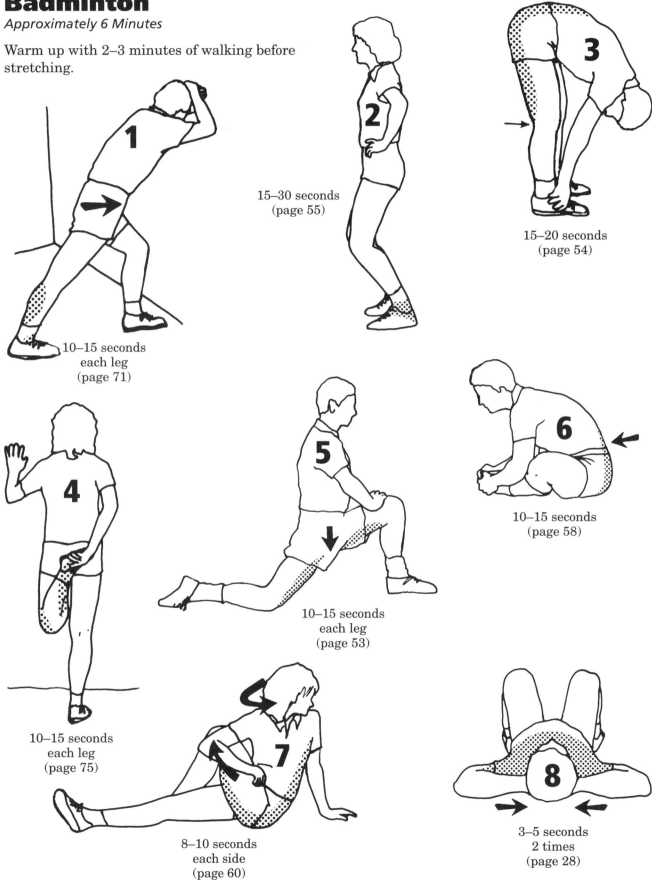

10–15 seconds
each leg
(page 71)

15–30 seconds
(page 55)

15–20 seconds
(page 54)

10–15 seconds
each leg
(page 75)

10–15 seconds
each leg
(page 53)

10–15 seconds
(page 58)

8–10 seconds
each side
(page 60)

3–5 seconds
2 times
(page 28)

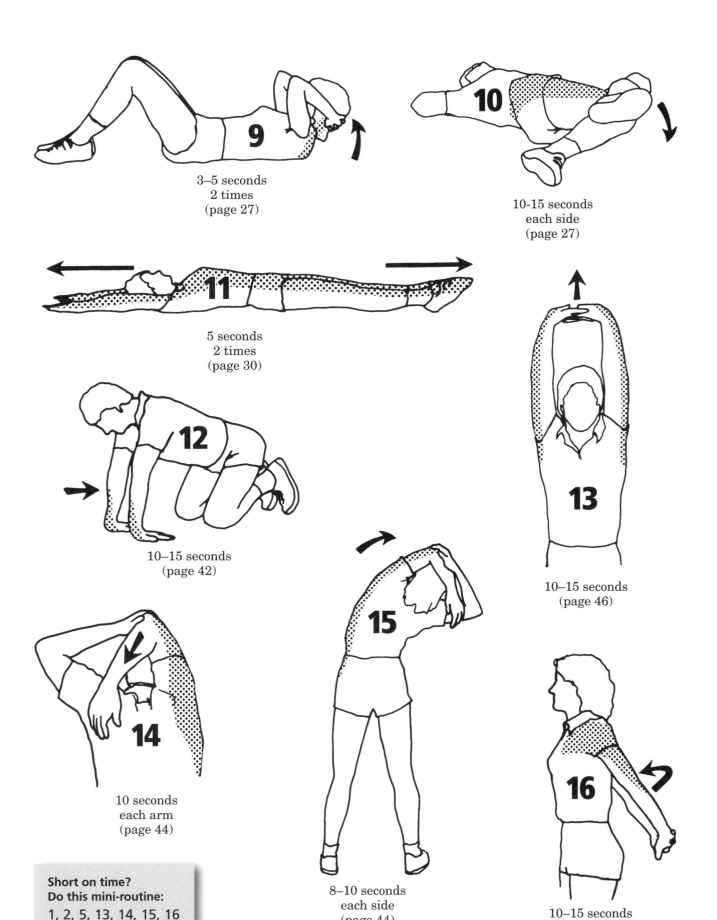

9
3–5 seconds
2 times
(page 27)

10
10-15 seconds
each side
(page 27)

11
5 seconds
2 times
(page 30)

12
10–15 seconds
(page 42)

13
10–15 seconds
(page 46)

14
10 seconds
each arm
(page 44)

15
8–10 seconds
each side
(page 44)

16
10–15 seconds
2 times
(page 44)

Short on time?
Do this mini-routine:
1, 2, 5, 13, 14, 15, 16
Approx. 3 minutes

Before and After
Baseball/Softball
Approximately 8 Minutes

Jog around the baseball field once before stretching.

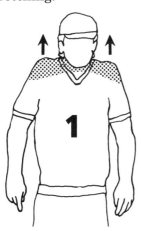

5 seconds
2–3 times
(page 46)

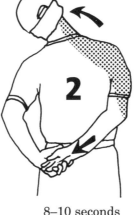

8–10 seconds
each arm
(page 47)

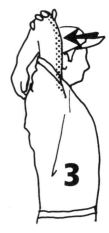

8–10 seconds
each arm
(page 44)

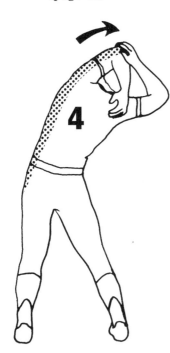

10 seconds
each side
(page 44)

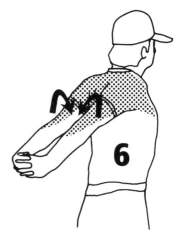

15 seconds
each arm
(page 43)

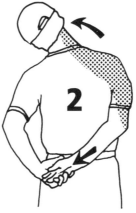

10–15 seconds
each arm
2 times
(page 47)

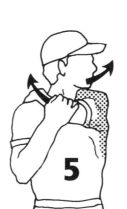

10–20 seconds
(page 43)

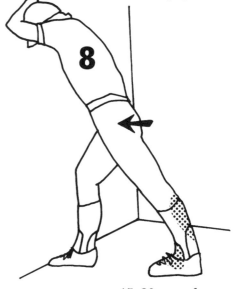

15–30 seconds
each leg
(page 71)

Stretching © 2000 by Bob and Jean Anderson. Shelter Publications, Inc.

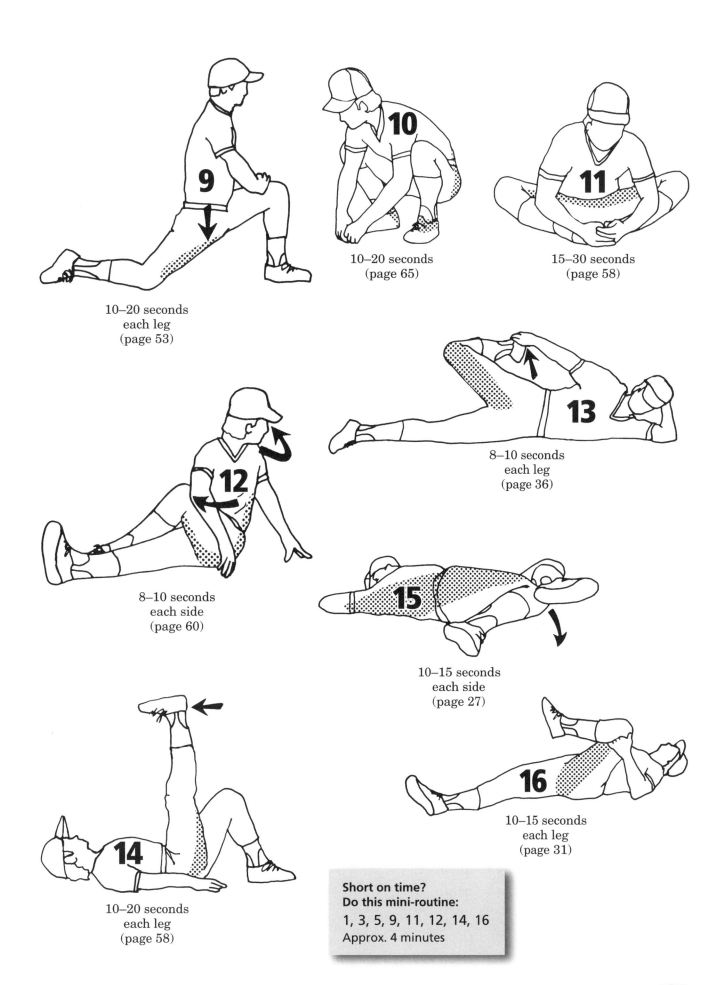

9

10–20 seconds
each leg
(page 53)

10

10–20 seconds
(page 65)

11

15–30 seconds
(page 58)

12

8–10 seconds
each side
(page 60)

13

8–10 seconds
each leg
(page 36)

15

10–15 seconds
each side
(page 27)

14

10–20 seconds
each leg
(page 58)

16

10–15 seconds
each leg
(page 31)

Short on time?
Do this mini-routine:
1, 3, 5, 9, 11, 12, 14, 16
Approx. 4 minutes

Before and After
Basketball
Approximately 7 Minutes

Warm up by jogging for 3–5 minutes before stretching.

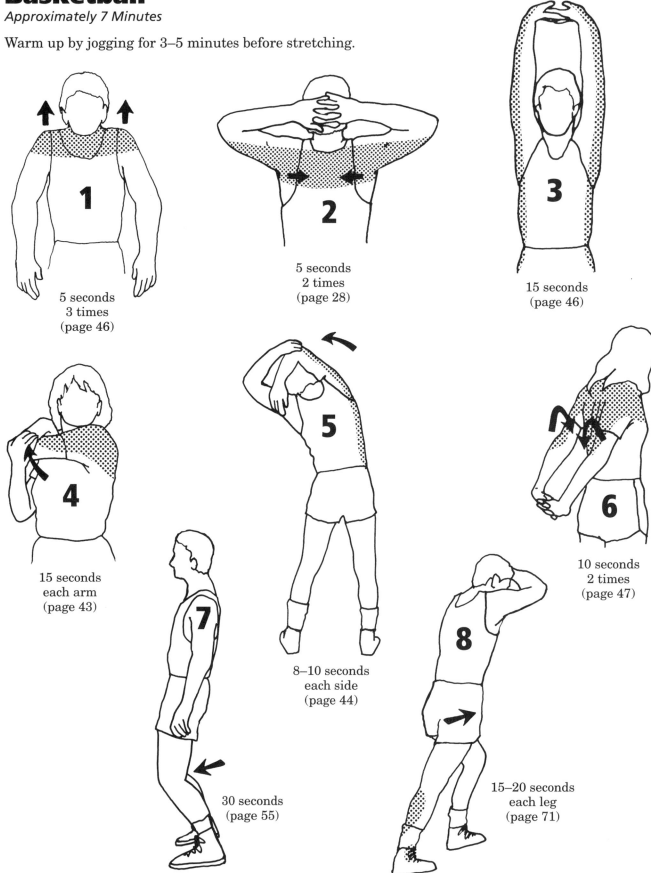

1

5 seconds
3 times
(page 46)

2

5 seconds
2 times
(page 28)

3

15 seconds
(page 46)

4

15 seconds
each arm
(page 43)

5

8–10 seconds
each side
(page 44)

6

10 seconds
2 times
(page 47)

7

30 seconds
(page 55)

8

15–20 seconds
each leg
(page 71)

Stretching © 2000 by Bob and Jean Anderson. Shelter Publications, Inc.

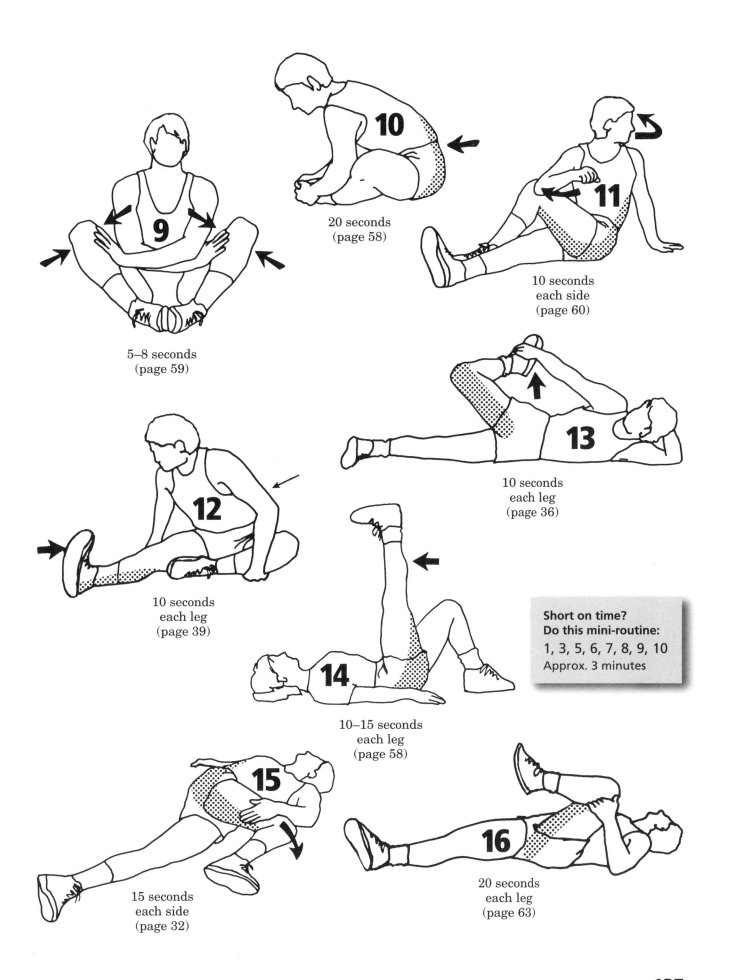

9

5–8 seconds
(page 59)

10

20 seconds
(page 58)

11

10 seconds
each side
(page 60)

12

10 seconds
each leg
(page 39)

13

10 seconds
each leg
(page 36)

14

10–15 seconds
each leg
(page 58)

Short on time?
Do this mini-routine:
1, 3, 5, 6, 7, 8, 9, 10
Approx. 3 minutes

15

15 seconds
each side
(page 32)

16

20 seconds
each leg
(page 63)

Bowling
Approximately 6 Minutes

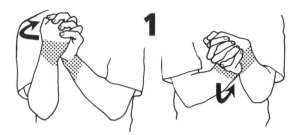

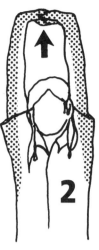

1

Rotate 10 times
each direction
(page 88)

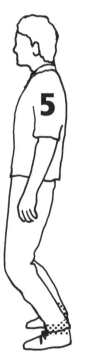

2

15 seconds
(page 46)

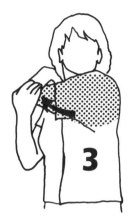

3

15 seconds
each arm
(page 43)

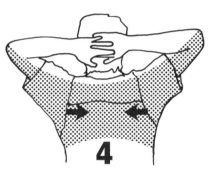

4

5 seconds
2 times
(page 91)

5

15–20 seconds
(page 55)

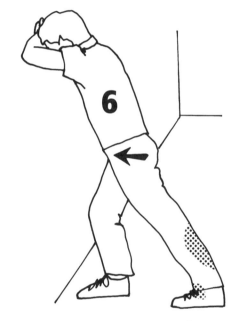

6

10–15 seconds
each leg
(page 71)

7

10 seconds
each leg
(page 51)

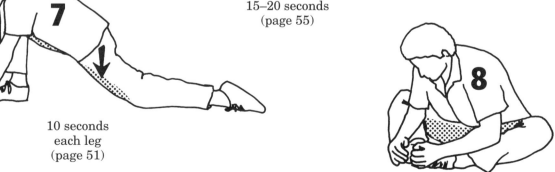

8

10 seconds
(page 58)

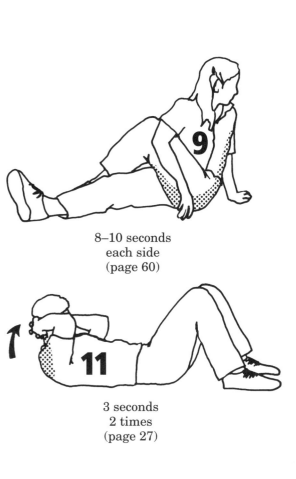

8–10 seconds
each side
(page 60)

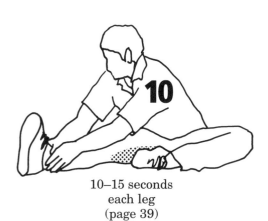

10

10–15 seconds
each leg
(page 39)

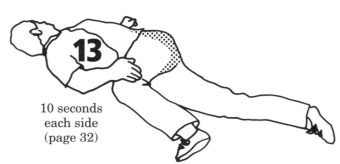

3 seconds
2 times
(page 27)

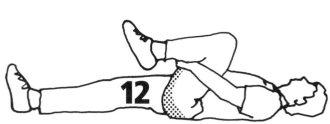

15–20 seconds
each leg
(page 31)

13

10 seconds
each side
(page 32)

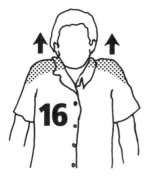

16

5 seconds
3 times
(page 46)

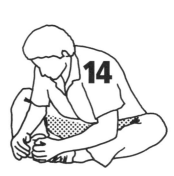

10 seconds
(page 58)

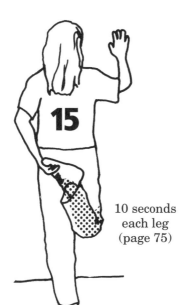

10 seconds
each leg
(page 75)

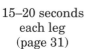

Short on time?
Do this mini-routine:
1, 2, 4, 5, 6, 7, 15
Approx. 2½ minutes

Before and After
Cycling
Approximately 8 Minutes

Walk for several minutes before stretching.

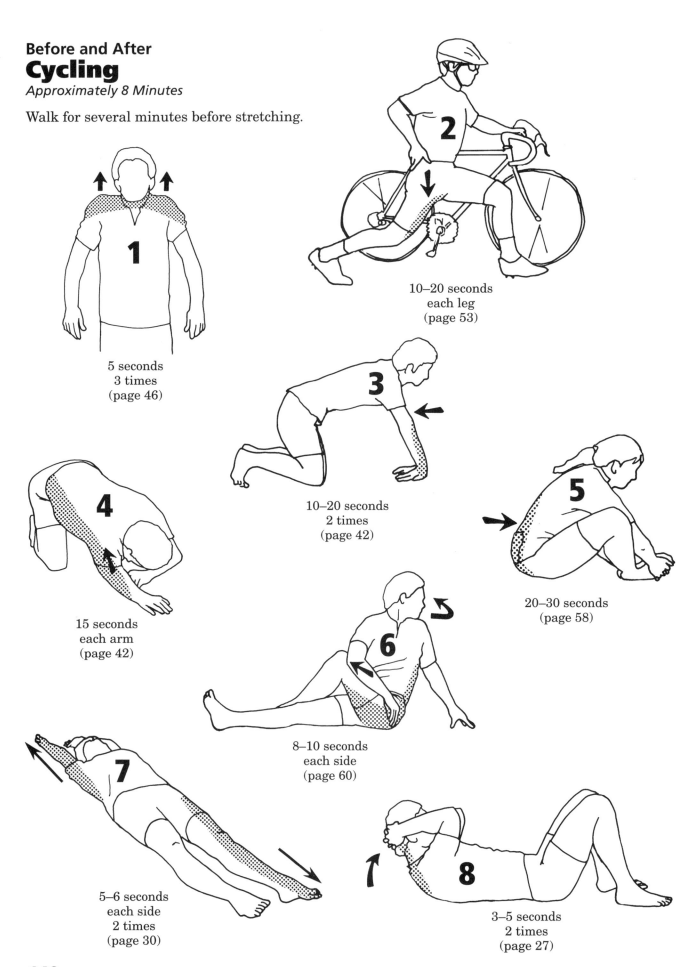

5 seconds
3 times
(page 46)

10–20 seconds
each leg
(page 53)

10–20 seconds
2 times
(page 42)

15 seconds
each arm
(page 42)

20–30 seconds
(page 58)

8–10 seconds
each side
(page 60)

5–6 seconds
each side
2 times
(page 30)

3–5 seconds
2 times
(page 27)

Stretching © 2000 by Bob and Jean Anderson. Shelter Publications, Inc.

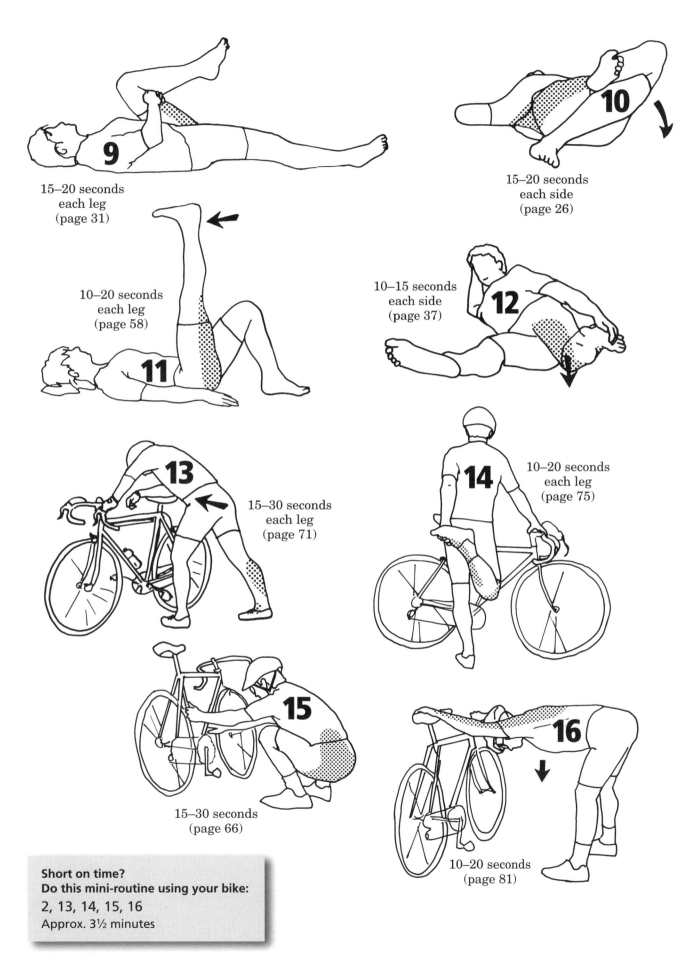

9
15–20 seconds
each leg
(page 31)

10
15–20 seconds
each side
(page 26)

11
10–20 seconds
each leg
(page 58)

12
10–15 seconds
each side
(page 37)

13
15–30 seconds
each leg
(page 71)

14
10–20 seconds
each leg
(page 75)

15
15–30 seconds
(page 66)

16
10–20 seconds
(page 81)

Short on time?
Do this mini-routine using your bike:
2, 13, 14, 15, 16
Approx. 3½ minutes

Before and After
Equestrian Sports
Approximately 5 Minutes

Walk for 2–3 minutes before stretching.

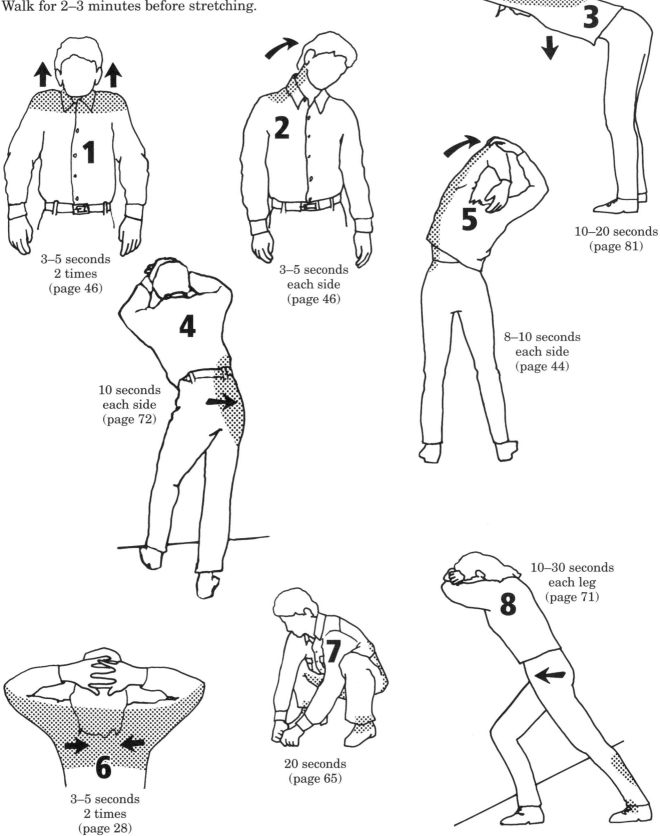

3–5 seconds
2 times
(page 46)

3–5 seconds
each side
(page 46)

10–20 seconds
(page 81)

10 seconds
each side
(page 72)

8–10 seconds
each side
(page 44)

10–30 seconds
each leg
(page 71)

3–5 seconds
2 times
(page 28)

20 seconds
(page 65)

Stretching © 2000 by Bob and Jean Anderson. Shelter Publications, Inc.

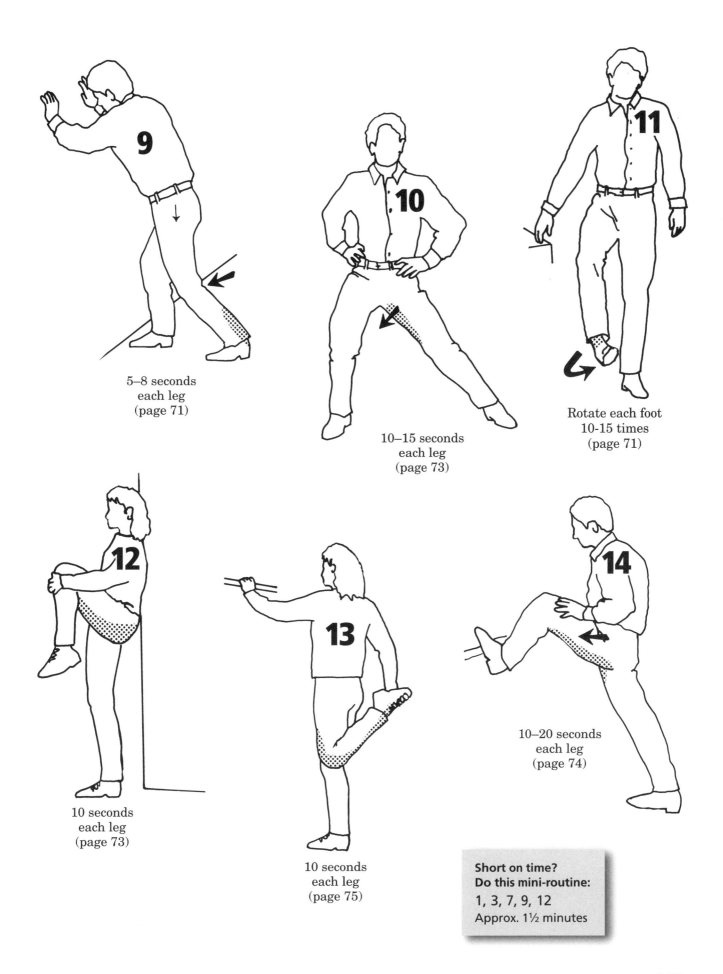

9

5–8 seconds
each leg
(page 71)

10

10–15 seconds
each leg
(page 73)

11

Rotate each foot
10-15 times
(page 71)

12

10 seconds
each leg
(page 73)

13

10 seconds
each leg
(page 75)

14

10–20 seconds
each leg
(page 74)

Short on time?
Do this mini-routine:
1, 3, 7, 9, 12
Approx. 1½ minutes

Before and After
Figure Skating
Approximately 8 Minutes

Warm up for 4–5 minutes before stretching.

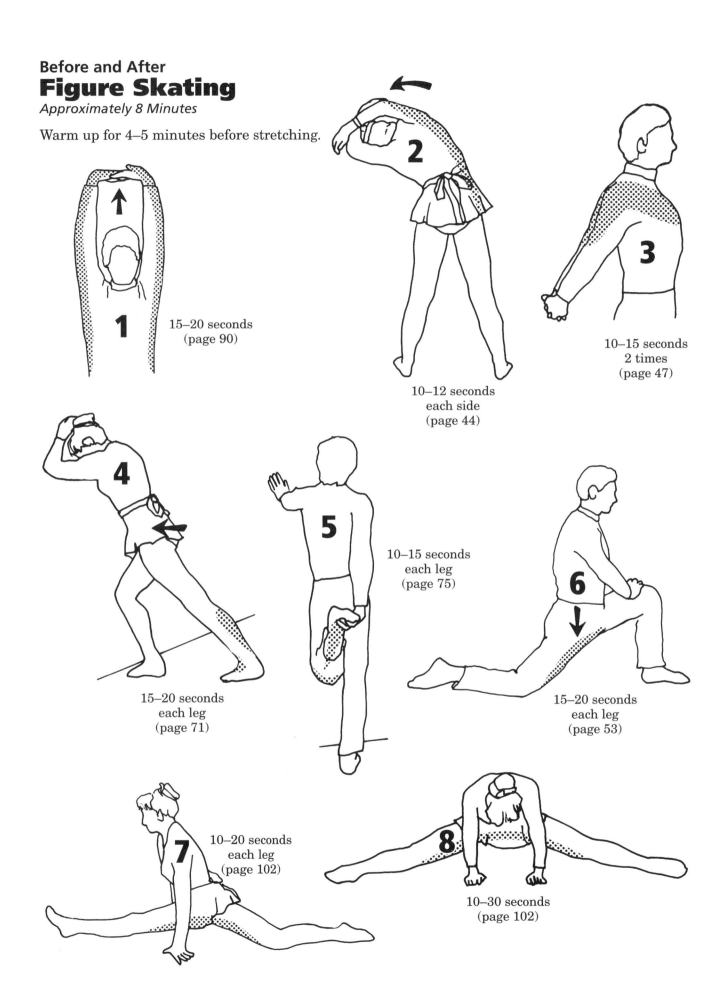

1 15–20 seconds
(page 90)

2 10–12 seconds
each side
(page 44)

3 10–15 seconds
2 times
(page 47)

4 15–20 seconds
each leg
(page 71)

5 10–15 seconds
each leg
(page 75)

6 15–20 seconds
each leg
(page 53)

7 10–20 seconds
each leg
(page 102)

8 10–30 seconds
(page 102)

Stretching © 2000 by Bob and Jean Anderson. Shelter Publications, Inc.

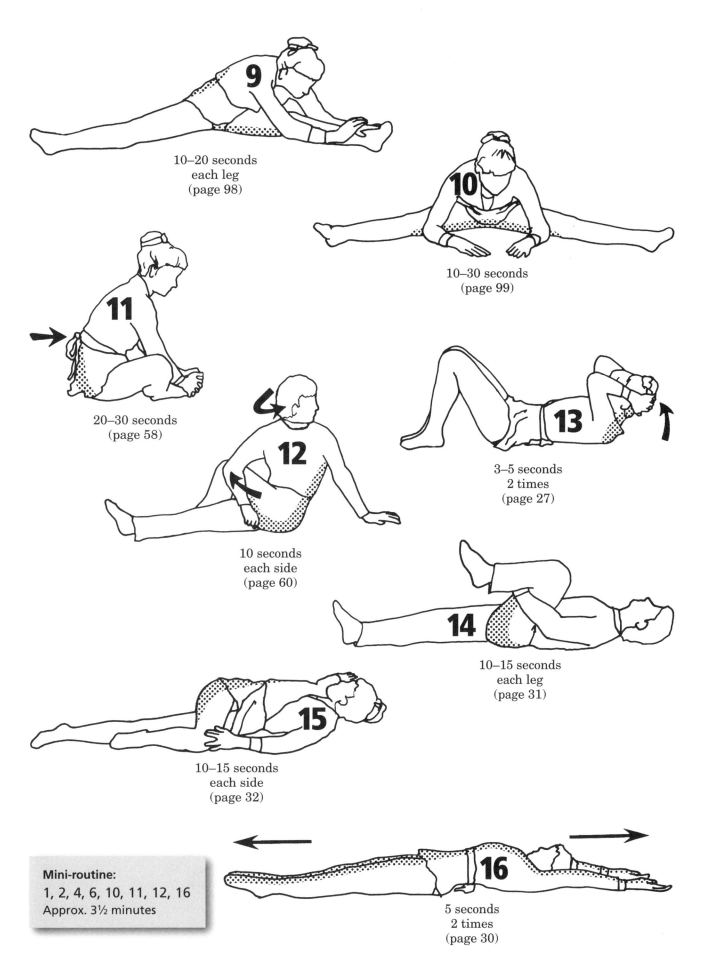

9
10–20 seconds
each leg
(page 98)

10
10–30 seconds
(page 99)

11
20–30 seconds
(page 58)

12
10 seconds
each side
(page 60)

13
3–5 seconds
2 times
(page 27)

14
10–15 seconds
each leg
(page 31)

15
10–15 seconds
each side
(page 32)

16
5 seconds
2 times
(page 30)

Mini-routine:
1, 2, 4, 6, 10, 11, 12, 16
Approx. 3½ minutes

Before and After
Football
Approximately 6 Minutes

Jog around the football field before stretching.

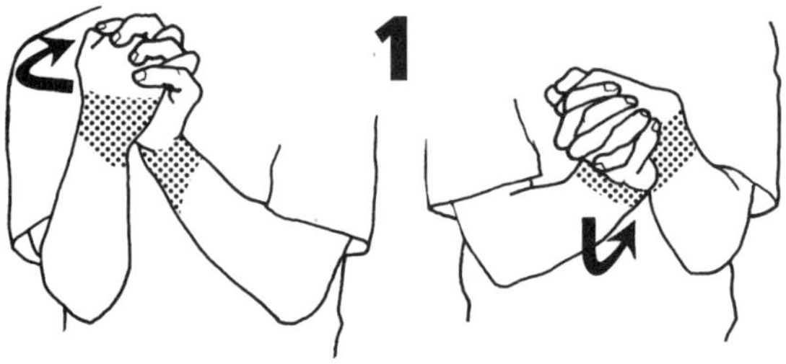

1

Rotate 10–15 times
each direction
(page 88)

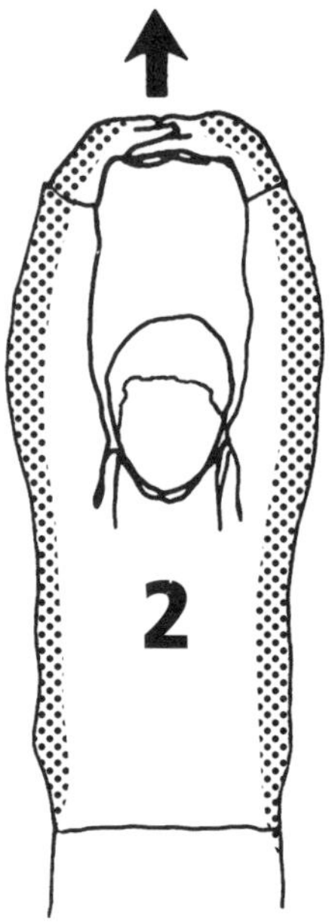

2

10 seconds
2 times
(page 46)

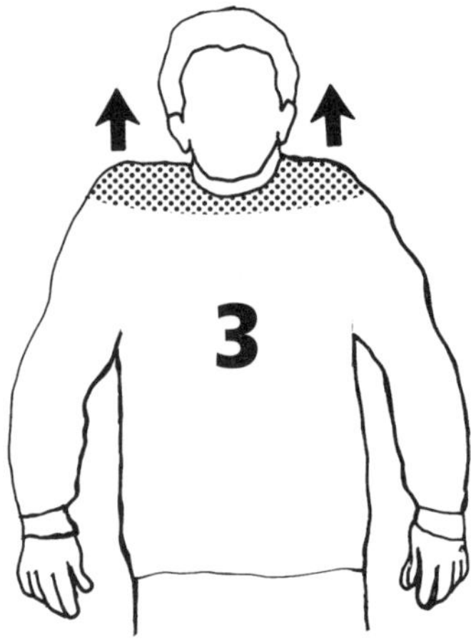

3

5 seconds
2 times
(page 46)

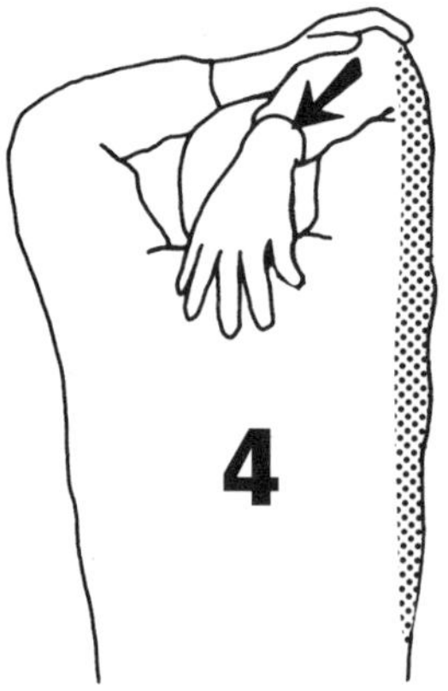

4

10–15 seconds
each arm
(page 44)

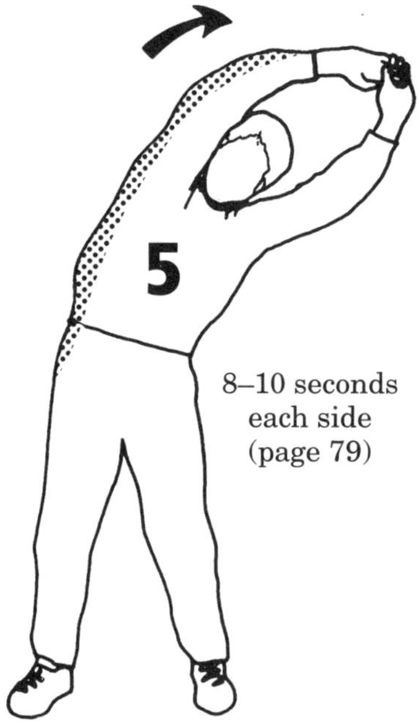

5

8–10 seconds
each side
(page 79)

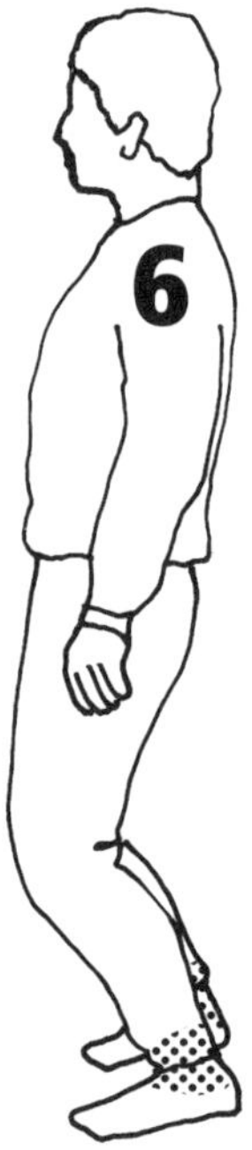

6

30 seconds
(page 59)

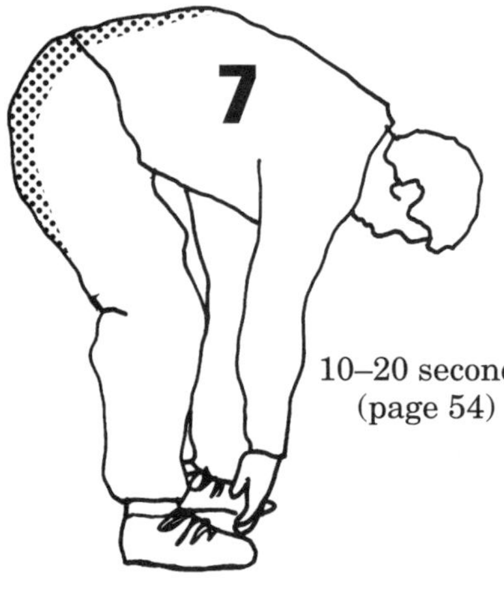

7

10–20 seconds
(page 54)

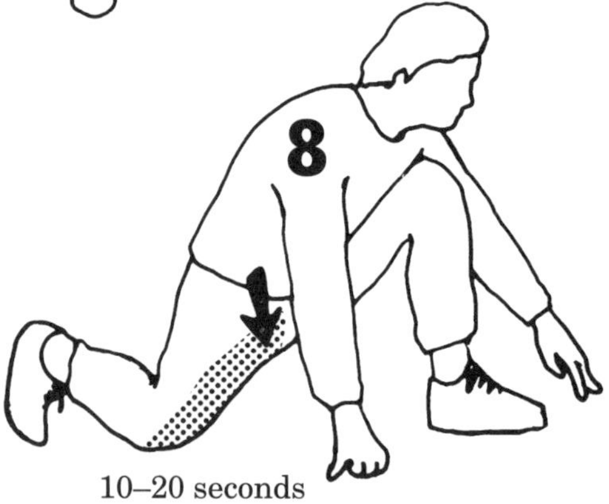

8

10–20 seconds
each leg
(page 51)

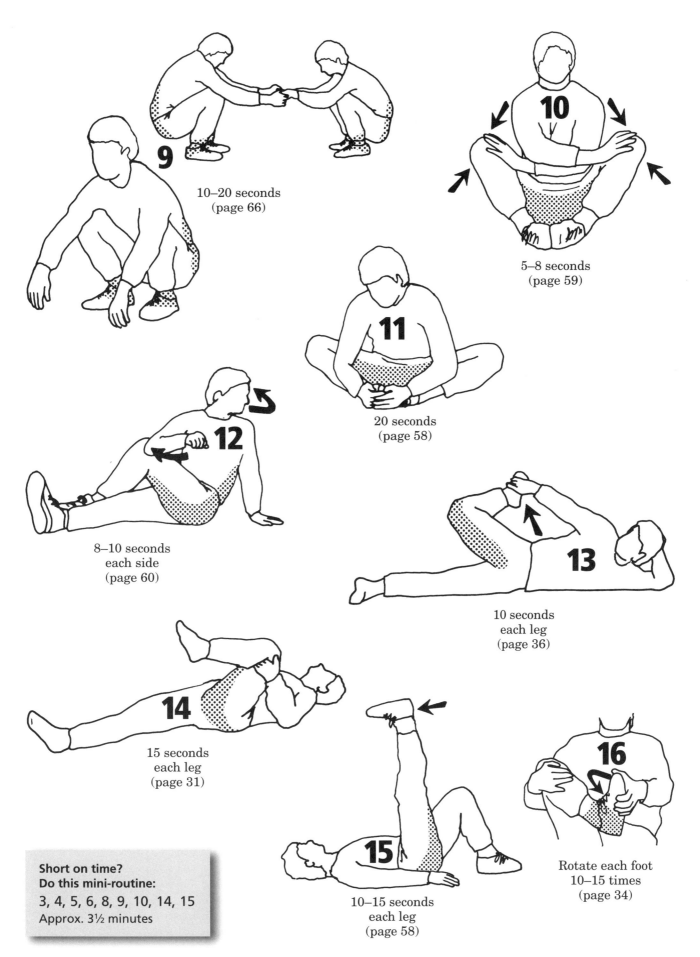

9
10–20 seconds
(page 66)

10
5–8 seconds
(page 59)

11
20 seconds
(page 58)

12
8–10 seconds
each side
(page 60)

13
10 seconds
each leg
(page 36)

14
15 seconds
each leg
(page 31)

15
10–15 seconds
each leg
(page 58)

16
Rotate each foot
10–15 times
(page 34)

Short on time?
Do this mini-routine:
3, 4, 5, 6, 8, 9, 10, 14, 15
Approx. 3½ minutes

Before and After
Golf
Approximately 6 Minutes

Walk for several minutes before stretching.

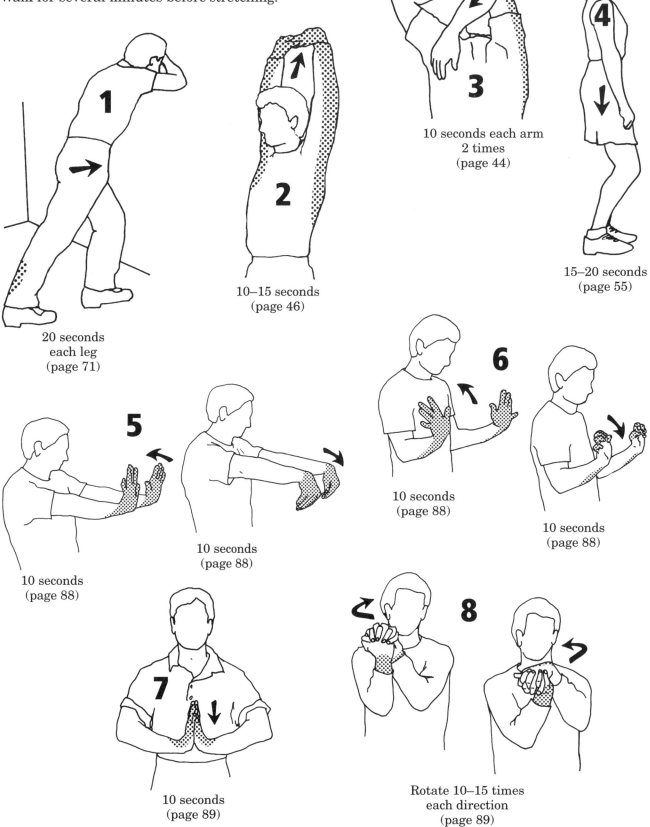

1

20 seconds
each leg
(page 71)

2

10–15 seconds
(page 46)

3

10 seconds each arm
2 times
(page 44)

4

15–20 seconds
(page 55)

5

10 seconds
(page 88)

10 seconds
(page 88)

6

10 seconds
(page 88)

10 seconds
(page 88)

7

10 seconds
(page 89)

8

Rotate 10–15 times
each direction
(page 89)

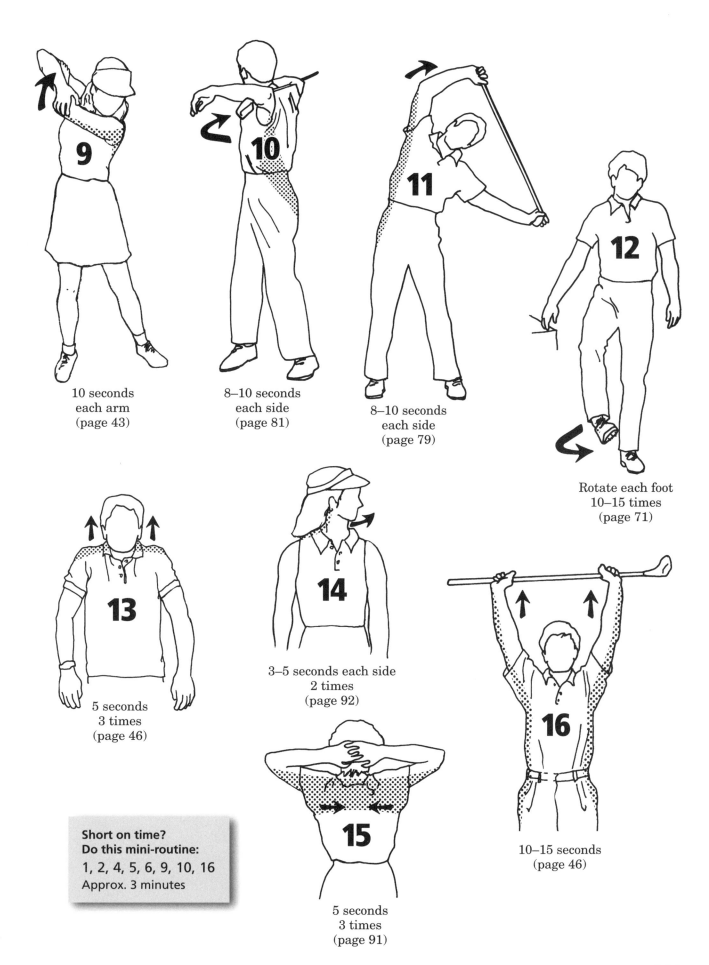

9

10 seconds
each arm
(page 43)

10

8–10 seconds
each side
(page 81)

11

8–10 seconds
each side
(page 79)

12

Rotate each foot
10–15 times
(page 71)

13

5 seconds
3 times
(page 46)

14

3–5 seconds each side
2 times
(page 92)

15

5 seconds
3 times
(page 91)

16

10–15 seconds
(page 46)

Short on time?
Do this mini-routine:
1, 2, 4, 5, 6, 9, 10, 16
Approx. 3 minutes

Before and After
Gymnastics
Approximately 8 Minutes

Warm up for 4–5 minutes by walking or jogging before stretching.

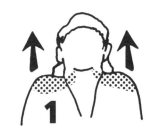

1

5 seconds
3 times
(page 46)

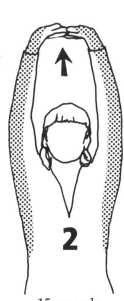

2

15 seconds
(page 46)

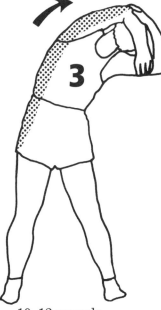

3

10–12 seconds
each side
(page 44)

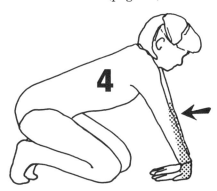

4

10–15 seconds
2 times
(page 42)

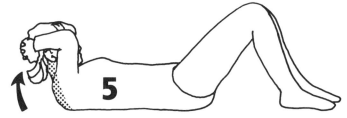

5

3–5 seconds
2 times
(page 27)

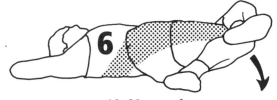

6

10–20 seconds
each side
(page 27)

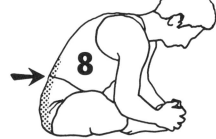

8

30 seconds
(page 65)

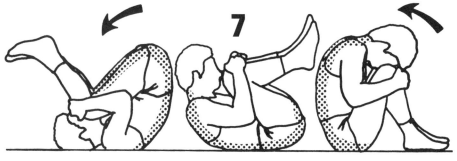

7

Gently roll
6–12 times
(page 63)

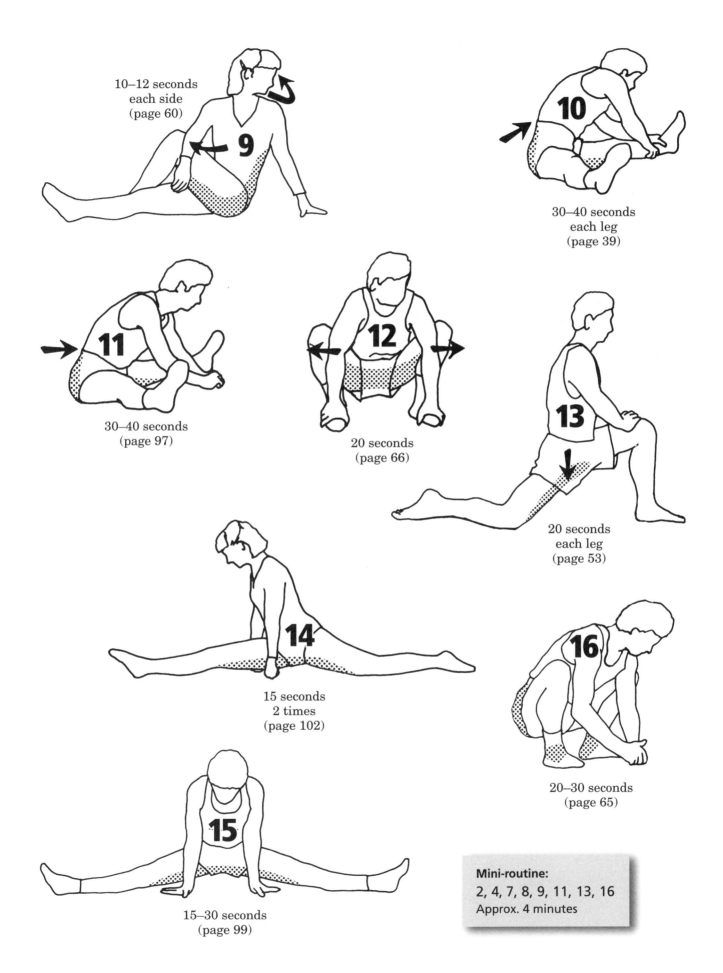

10–12 seconds
each side
(page 60)

9

10

30–40 seconds
each leg
(page 39)

11

30–40 seconds
(page 97)

12

20 seconds
(page 66)

13

20 seconds
each leg
(page 53)

14

15 seconds
2 times
(page 102)

16

20–30 seconds
(page 65)

15

15–30 seconds
(page 99)

Mini-routine:
2, 4, 7, 8, 9, 11, 13, 16
Approx. 4 minutes

Before, During Breaks, and After

Hiking

Approximately 7 Minutes

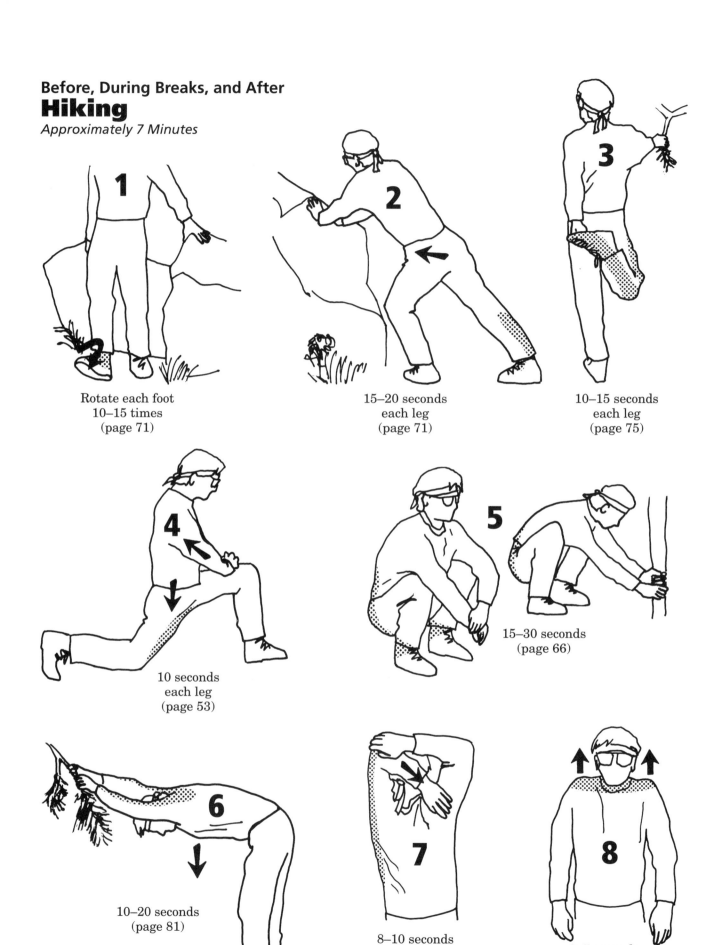

Rotate each foot
10–15 times
(page 71)

15–20 seconds
each leg
(page 71)

10–15 seconds
each leg
(page 75)

10 seconds
each leg
(page 53)

15–30 seconds
(page 66)

10–20 seconds
(page 81)

8–10 seconds
each arm
(page 44)

3–5 seconds
several times
(page 46)

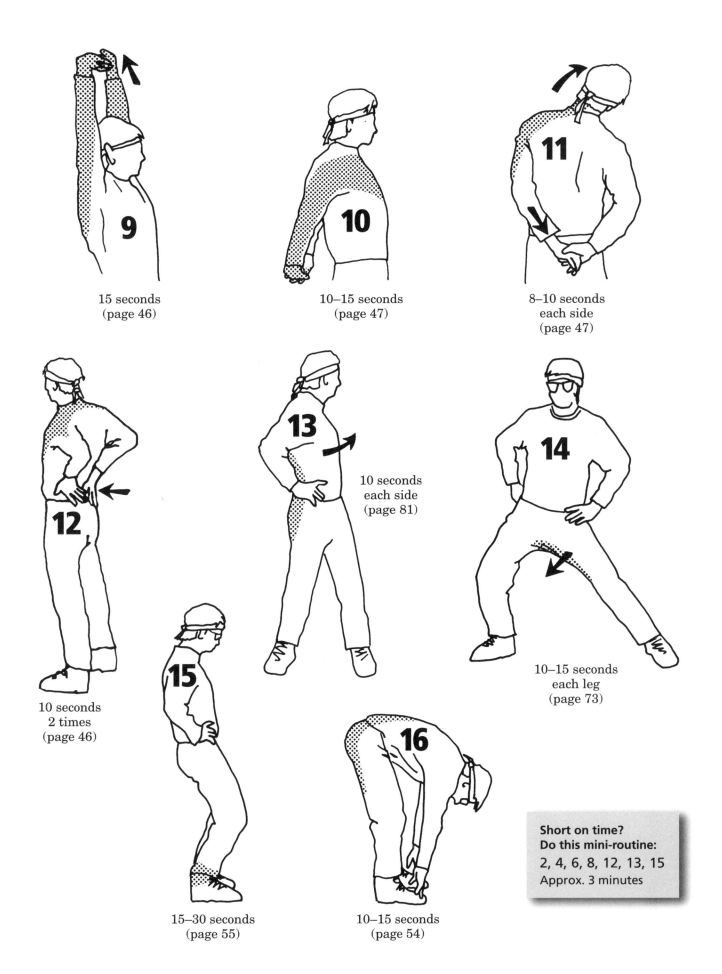

9

15 seconds
(page 46)

10

10–15 seconds
(page 47)

11

8–10 seconds
each side
(page 47)

12

10 seconds
2 times
(page 46)

13

10 seconds
each side
(page 81)

14

10–15 seconds
each leg
(page 73)

15

15–30 seconds
(page 55)

16

10–15 seconds
(page 54)

**Short on time?
Do this mini-routine:**
2, 4, 6, 8, 12, 13, 15
Approx. 3 minutes

Before and After
Ice Hockey
Approximately 8 Minutes

Warm up by walking or riding a stationary bike for 2–4 minutes before stretching.

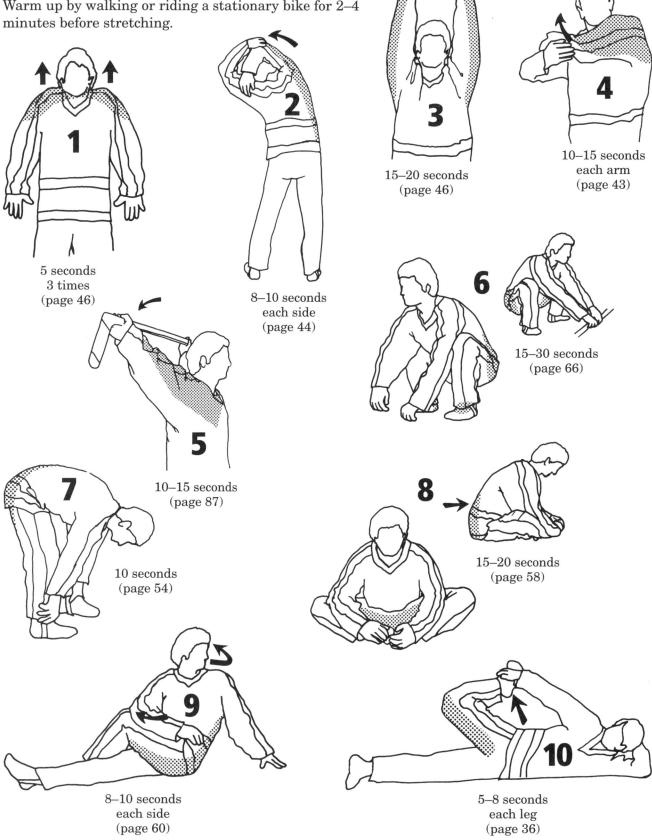

1 5 seconds
3 times
(page 46)

2 8–10 seconds
each side
(page 44)

3 15–20 seconds
(page 46)

4 10–15 seconds
each arm
(page 43)

5 10–15 seconds
(page 87)

6 15–30 seconds
(page 66)

7 10 seconds
(page 54)

8 15–20 seconds
(page 58)

9 8–10 seconds
each side
(page 60)

10 5–8 seconds
each leg
(page 36)

Stretching © 2000 by Bob and Jean Anderson. Shelter Publications, Inc.

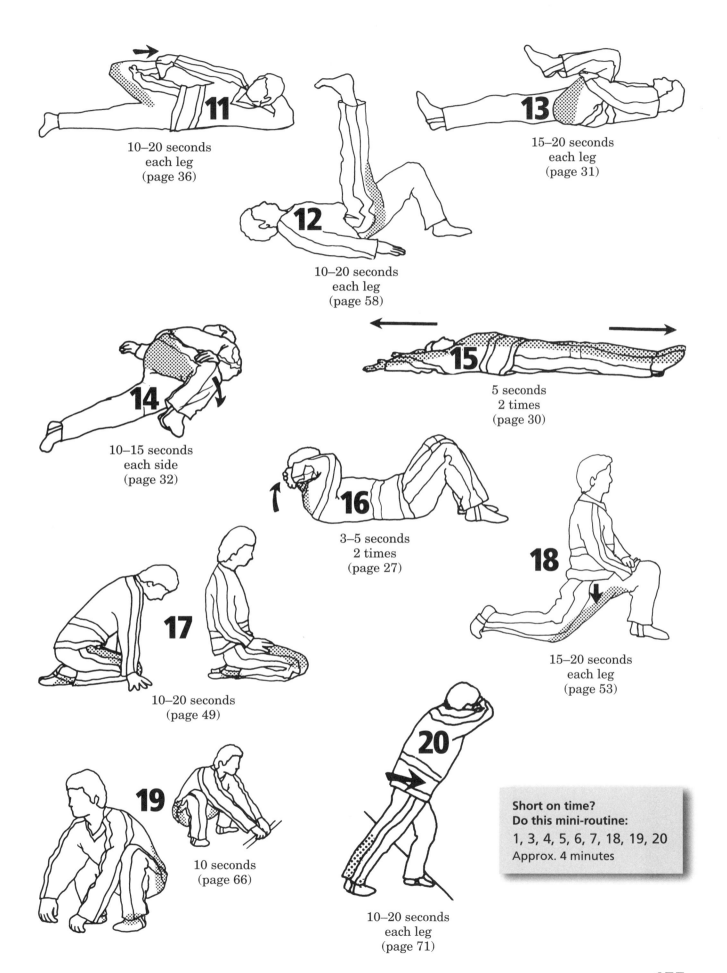

11
10–20 seconds
each leg
(page 36)

12
10–20 seconds
each leg
(page 58)

13
15–20 seconds
each leg
(page 31)

14
10–15 seconds
each side
(page 32)

15
5 seconds
2 times
(page 30)

16
3–5 seconds
2 times
(page 27)

17
10–20 seconds
(page 49)

18
15–20 seconds
each leg
(page 53)

19
10 seconds
(page 66)

20
10–20 seconds
each leg
(page 71)

Short on time?
Do this mini-routine:
1, 3, 4, 5, 6, 7, 18, 19, 20
Approx. 4 minutes

Walk for several minutes before stretching.

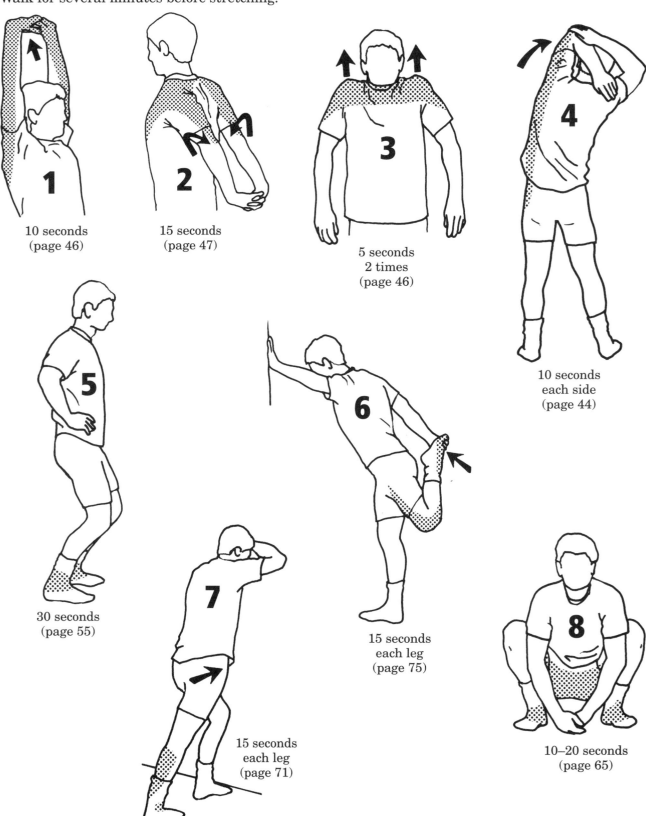

10 seconds
(page 46)

15 seconds
(page 47)

5 seconds
2 times
(page 46)

10 seconds
each side
(page 44)

30 seconds
(page 55)

15 seconds
each leg
(page 75)

15 seconds
each leg
(page 71)

10–20 seconds
(page 65)

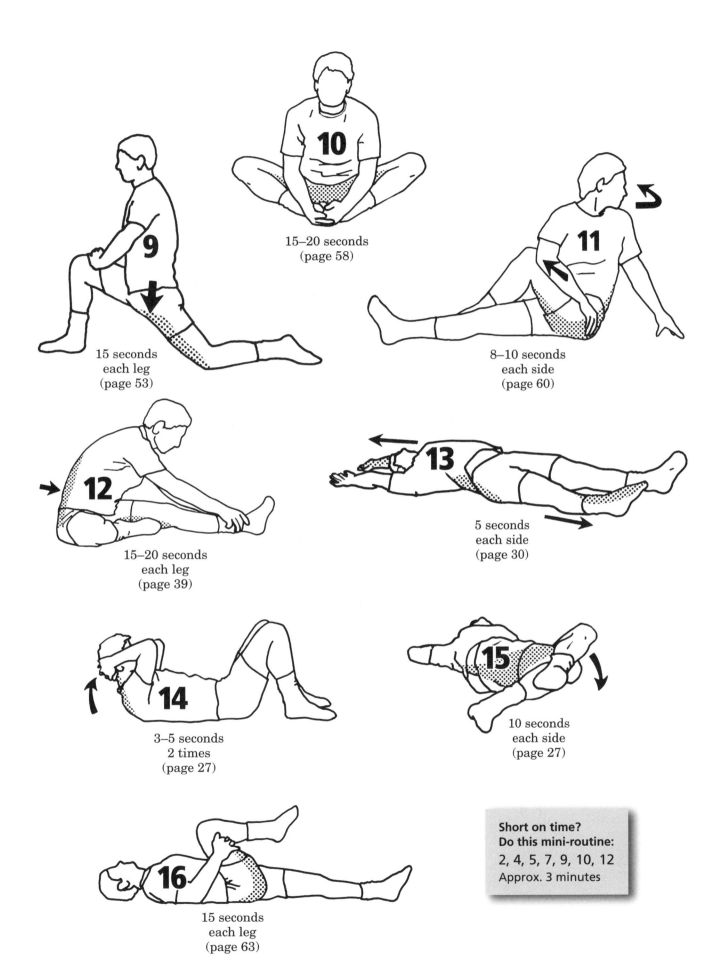

9

15 seconds
each leg
(page 53)

10

15–20 seconds
(page 58)

11

8–10 seconds
each side
(page 60)

12

15–20 seconds
each leg
(page 39)

13

5 seconds
each side
(page 30)

14

3–5 seconds
2 times
(page 27)

15

10 seconds
each side
(page 27)

16

15 seconds
each leg
(page 63)

Short on time?
Do this mini-routine:
2, 4, 5, 7, 9, 10, 12
Approx. 3 minutes

Before and After
Kayaking
Approximately 7 Minutes

Walk for several minutes before stretching.

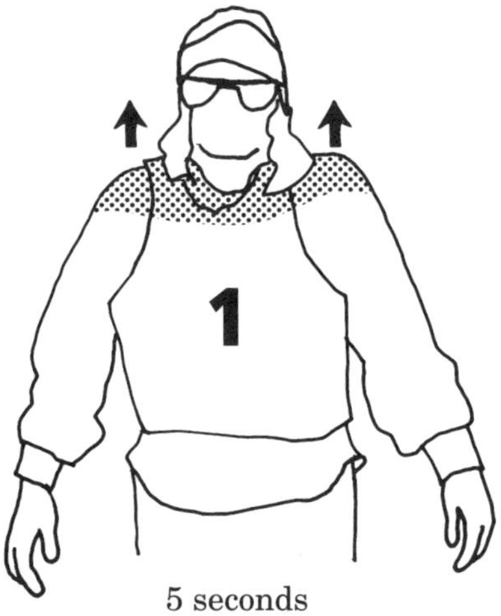

1

5 seconds
3 times
(page 46)

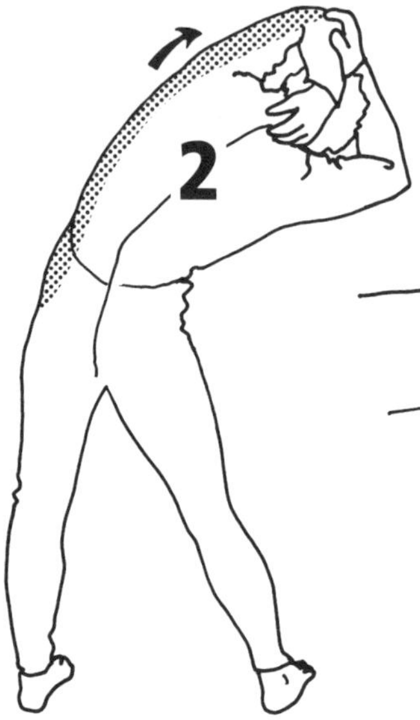

2

10 seconds
each side
(page 44)

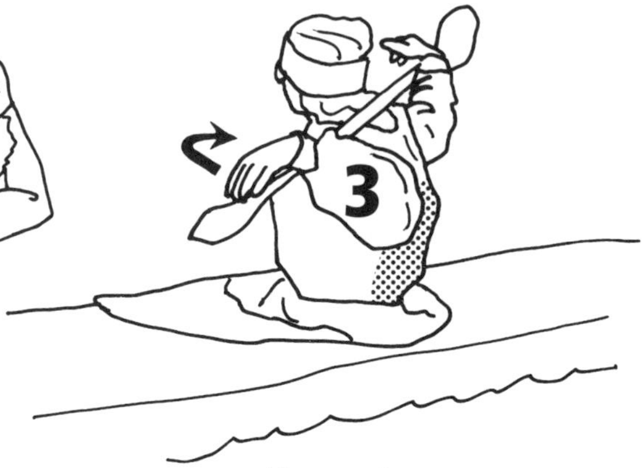

3

10 seconds
each side
(page 81)

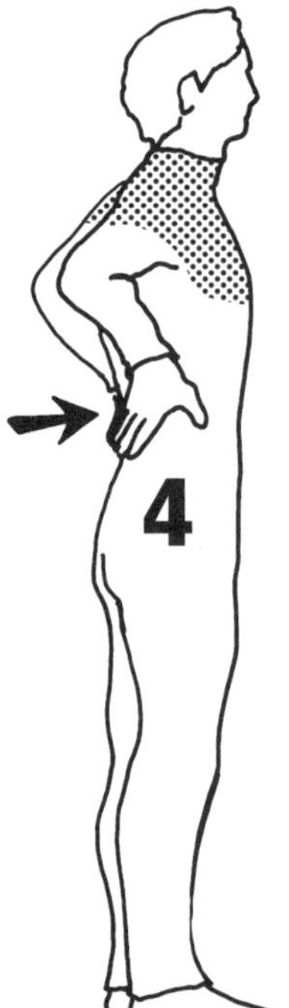

4

10 seconds
(page 46)

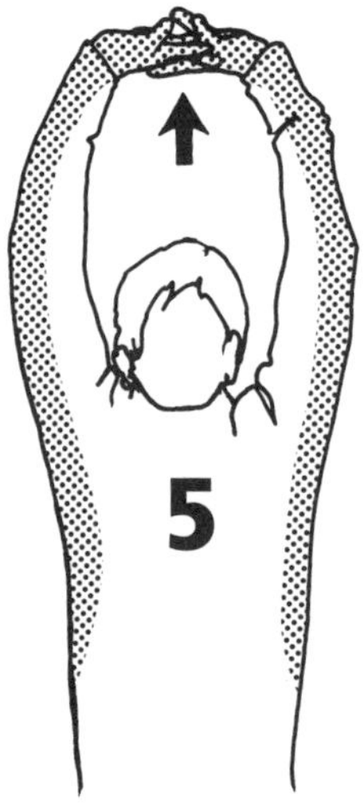

5

15 seconds
(page 46)

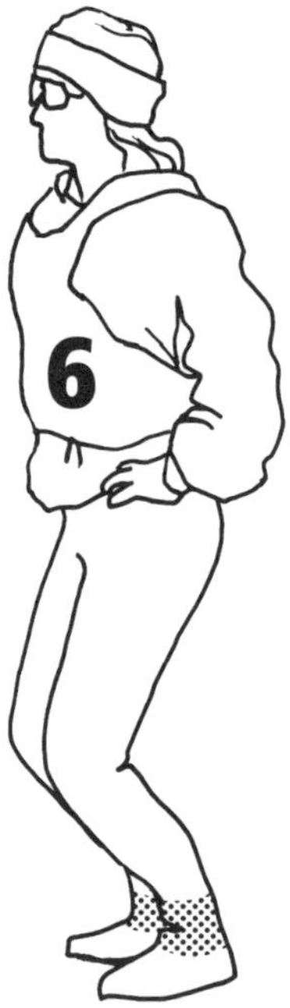

6

30 seconds
(page 55)

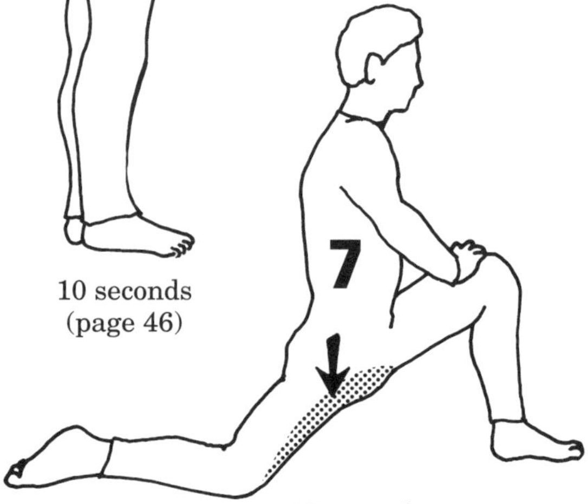

7

15 seconds
each leg
(page 53)

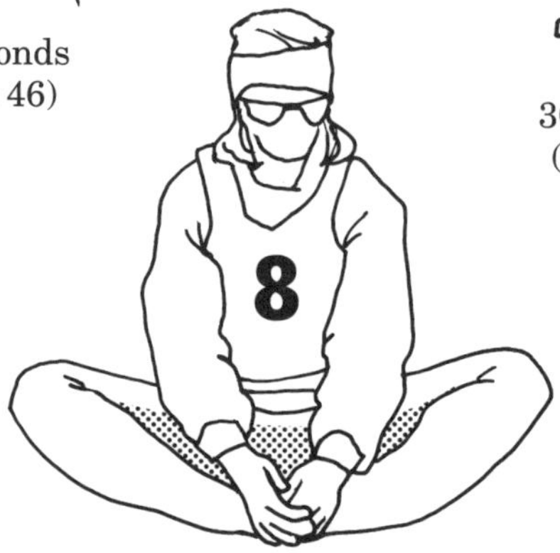

8

15–20 seconds
(page 58)

Stretching © 2000 by Bob and Jean Anderson. Shelter Publications, Inc.

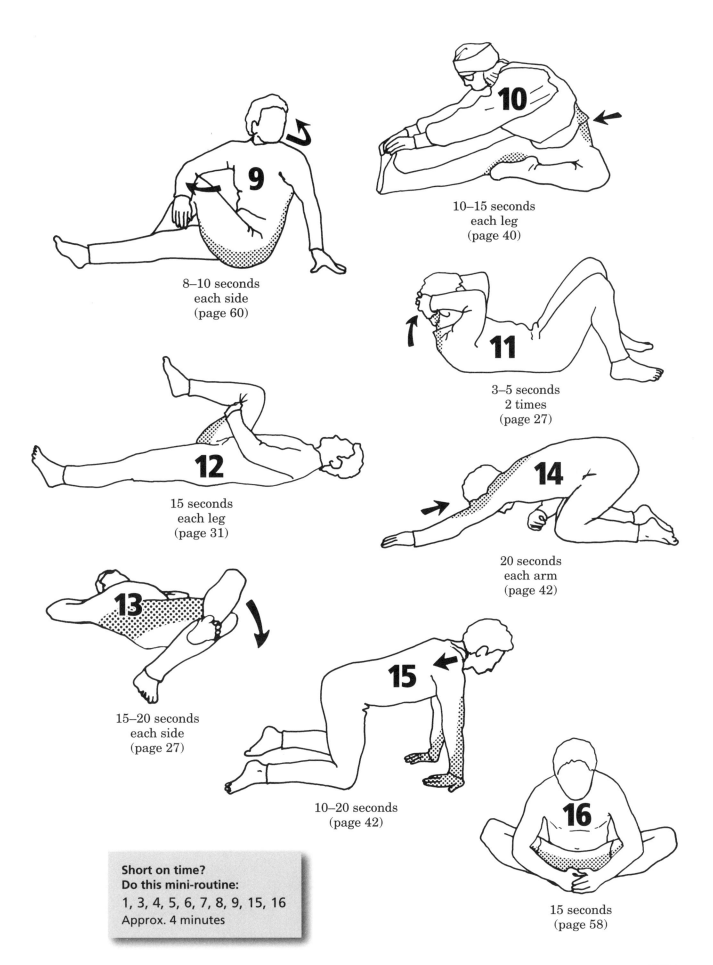

9

8–10 seconds
each side
(page 60)

10

10–15 seconds
each leg
(page 40)

11

3–5 seconds
2 times
(page 27)

12

15 seconds
each leg
(page 31)

14

20 seconds
each arm
(page 42)

13

15–20 seconds
each side
(page 27)

15

10–20 seconds
(page 42)

16

15 seconds
(page 58)

Short on time?
Do this mini-routine:
1, 3, 4, 5, 6, 7, 8, 9, 15, 16
Approx. 4 minutes

Before and After
Martial Arts
Approximately 7 Minutes

Note: These stretches are not intended to replace your traditional routine, but can be used for improvement of overall flexibility. They should be preceded by a good warm-up.

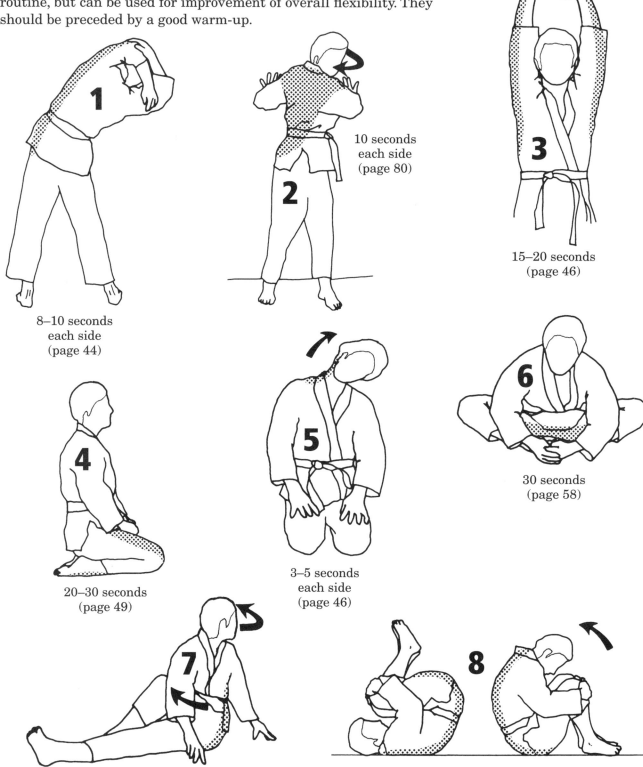

8–10 seconds
each side
(page 44)

10 seconds
each side
(page 80)

15–20 seconds
(page 46)

20–30 seconds
(page 49)

3–5 seconds
each side
(page 46)

30 seconds
(page 58)

10 seconds
each side
(page 60)

Roll back and forth
10–12 times
(page 63)

Stretching © 2000 by Bob and Jean Anderson. Shelter Publications, Inc.

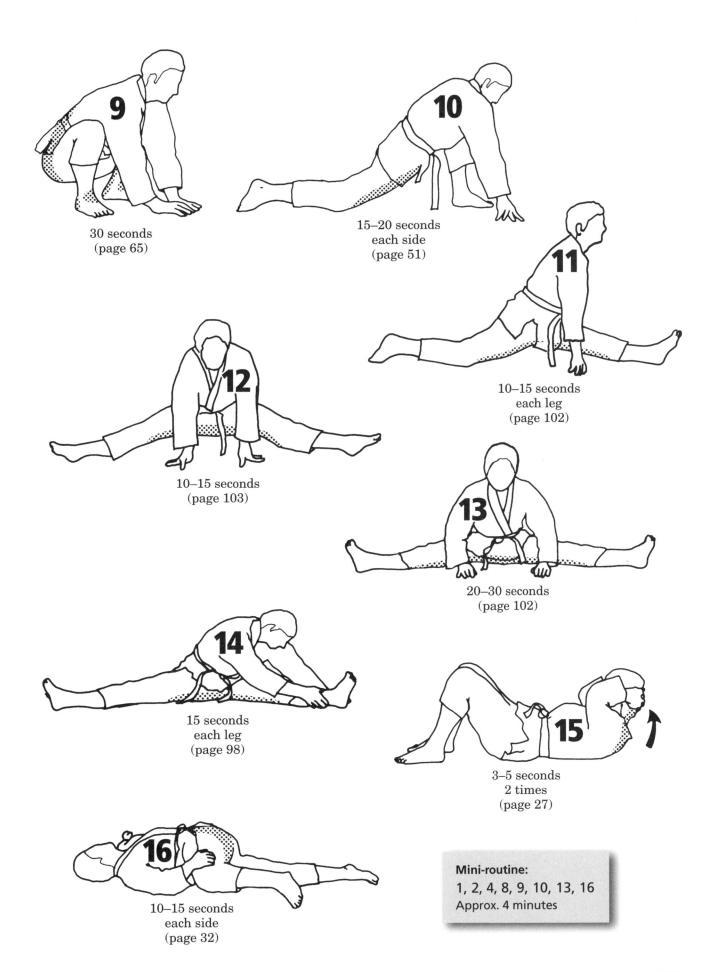

9
30 seconds
(page 65)

10
15–20 seconds
each side
(page 51)

11
10–15 seconds
each leg
(page 102)

12
10–15 seconds
(page 103)

13
20–30 seconds
(page 102)

14
15 seconds
each leg
(page 98)

15
3–5 seconds
2 times
(page 27)

16
10–15 seconds
each side
(page 32)

Mini-routine:
1, 2, 4, 8, 9, 10, 13, 16
Approx. 4 minutes

Before and After
Motocross
Approximately 6 Minutes

Walk around for several minutes before stretching.

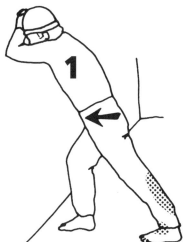

1

15 seconds
each leg
(page 71)

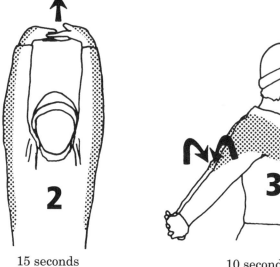

2

15 seconds
(page 46)

3

10 seconds
(page 47)

4

8–10 seconds
each side
(page 44)

5

10 seconds
(page 49)

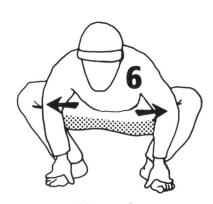

6

10 seconds
(page 66)

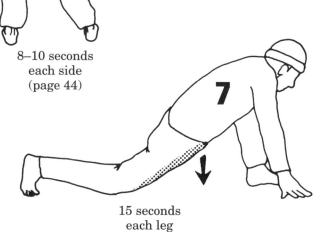

7

15 seconds
each leg
(page 52)

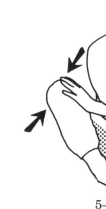

8

5–6 seconds
(page 59)

Stretching © 2000 by Bob and Jean Anderson. Shelter Publications, Inc.

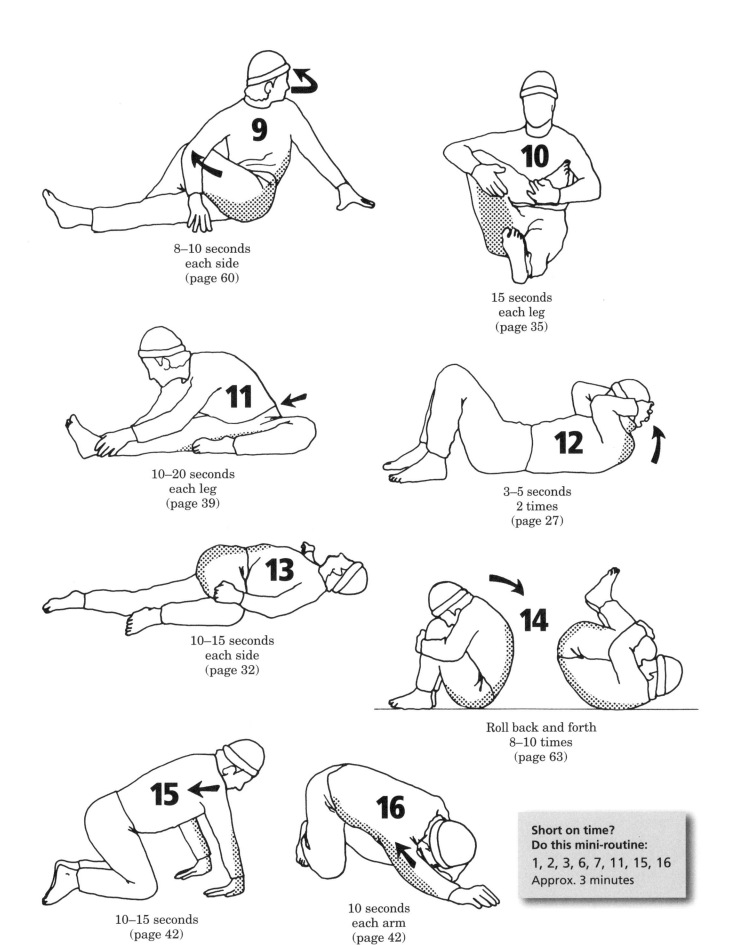

9

8–10 seconds
each side
(page 60)

10

15 seconds
each leg
(page 35)

11

10–20 seconds
each leg
(page 39)

12

3–5 seconds
2 times
(page 27)

13

10–15 seconds
each side
(page 32)

14

Roll back and forth
8–10 times
(page 63)

15

10–15 seconds
(page 42)

16

10 seconds
each arm
(page 42)

Short on time?
Do this mini-routine:
1, 2, 3, 6, 7, 11, 15, 16
Approx. 3 minutes

Before and After
Mountain Biking
Approximately 6 Minutes

Warm up by riding or walking for
3–5 minutes before stretching.

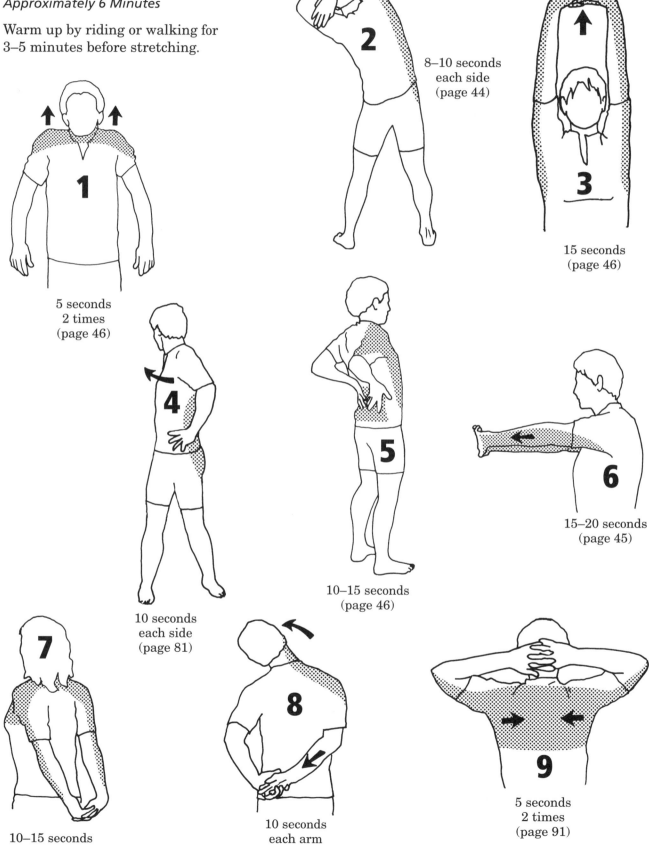

5 seconds
2 times
(page 46)

8–10 seconds
each side
(page 44)

15 seconds
(page 46)

10 seconds
each side
(page 81)

10–15 seconds
(page 46)

15–20 seconds
(page 45)

10–15 seconds
(page 47)

10 seconds
each arm
(page 47)

5 seconds
2 times
(page 91)

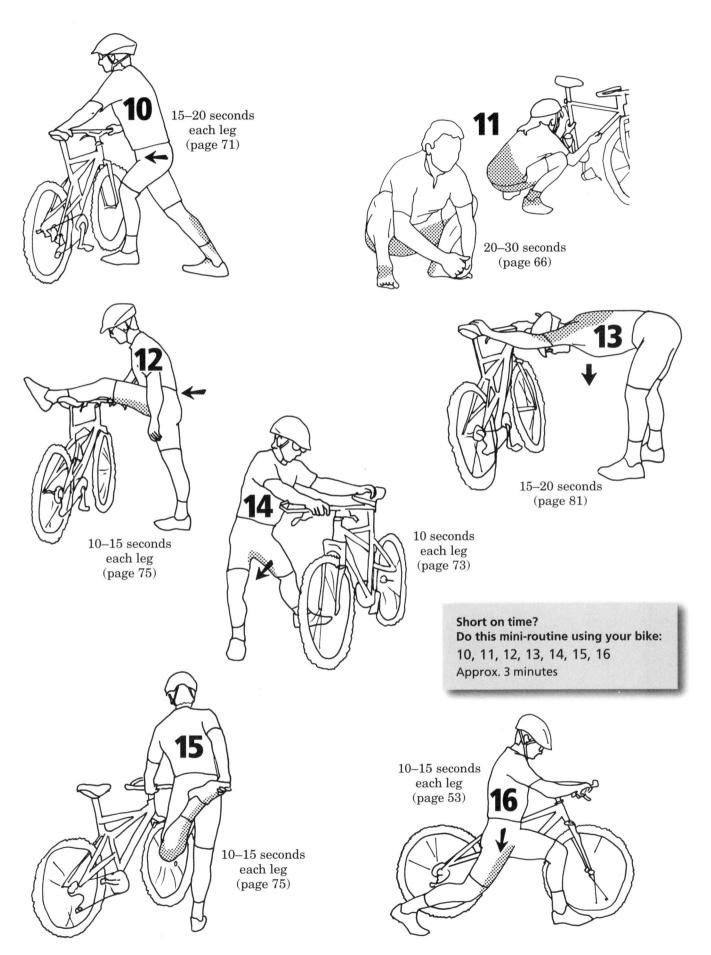

10 15–20 seconds
each leg
(page 71)

11 20–30 seconds
(page 66)

12 10–15 seconds
each leg
(page 75)

13 15–20 seconds
(page 81)

14 10 seconds
each leg
(page 73)

Short on time?
Do this mini-routine using your bike:
10, 11, 12, 13, 14, 15, 16
Approx. 3 minutes

15 10–15 seconds
each leg
(page 75)

16 10–15 seconds
each leg
(page 53)

Before and After
Racquetball, Handball & Squash
Approximately 7 Minutes

Warm up for 2–4 minutes before stretching.

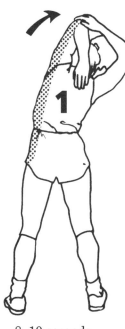

1

8–10 seconds
each side
(page 44)

2

10 seconds
each arm
(page 47)

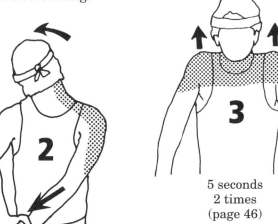

3

5 seconds
2 times
(page 46)

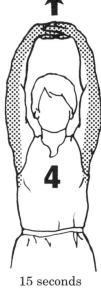

4

15 seconds
(page 46)

5

10 seconds
each arm
(page 82)

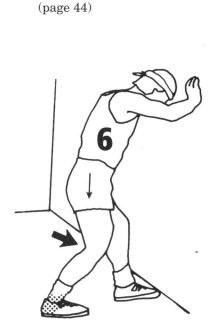

6

10 seconds
each leg
(page 71)

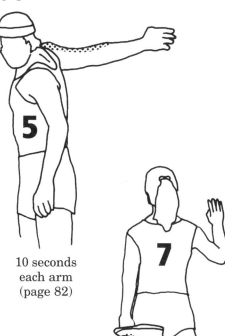

7

10–15 seconds
each leg
(page 75)

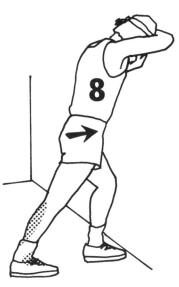

8

10–20 seconds
each leg
(page 71)

Stretching © 2000 by Bob and Jean Anderson. Shelter Publications, Inc.

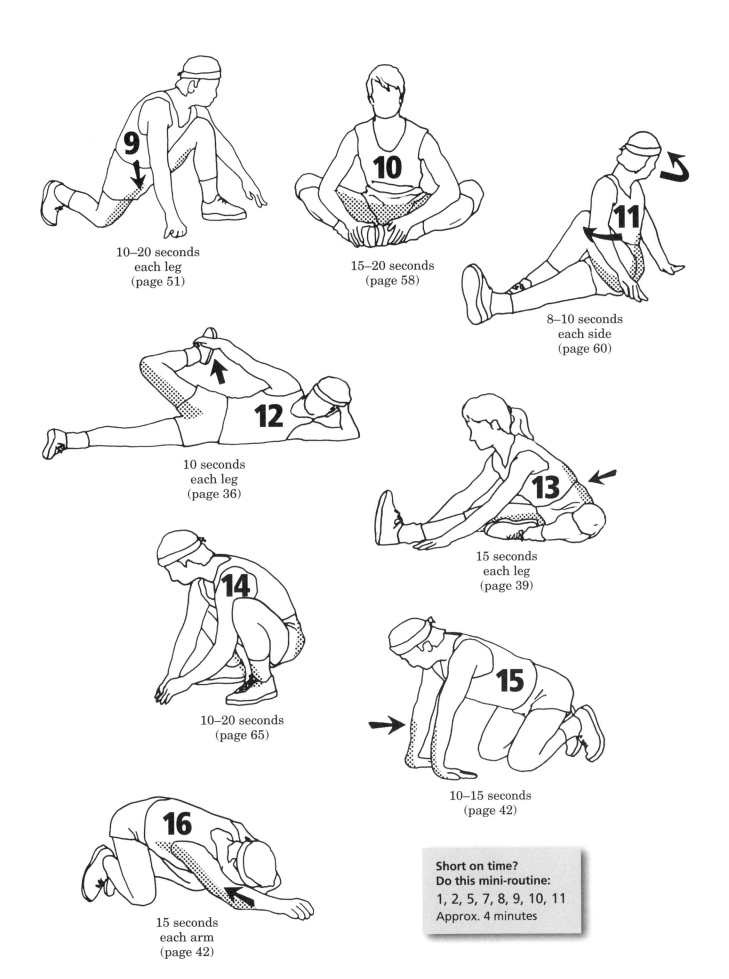

9 10–20 seconds
each leg
(page 51)

10 15–20 seconds
(page 58)

11 8–10 seconds
each side
(page 60)

12 10 seconds
each leg
(page 36)

13 15 seconds
each leg
(page 39)

14 10–20 seconds
(page 65)

15 10–15 seconds
(page 42)

16 15 seconds
each arm
(page 42)

Short on time?
Do this mini-routine:
1, 2, 5, 7, 8, 9, 10, 11
Approx. 4 minutes

Before and After
Rock Climbing
Approximately 6 Minutes

Walk for several minutes before stretching.

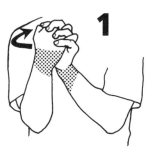

1

Rotate wrists
10 times clockwise and
counterclockwise
(page 88)

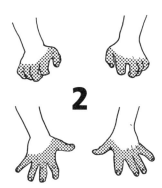

2

10 seconds each position
2 times
(page 88)

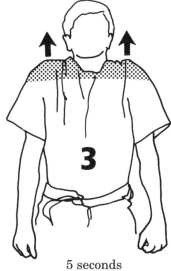

3

5 seconds
3 times
(page 46)

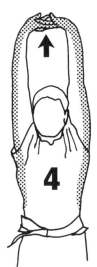

4

15 seconds
(page 46)

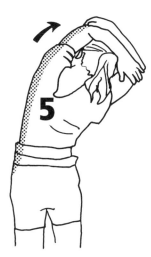

5

10 seconds
each side
(page 44)

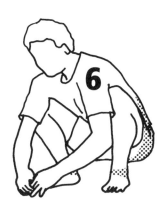

6

15–30 seconds
(page 65)

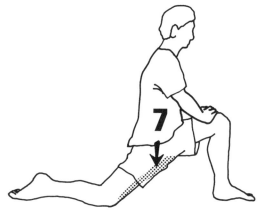

7

15 seconds
each leg
(page 53)

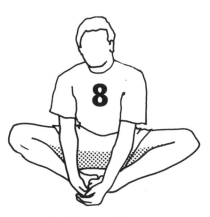

8

15–30 seconds
(page 58)

Stretching © 2000 by Bob and Jean Anderson. Shelter Publications, Inc.

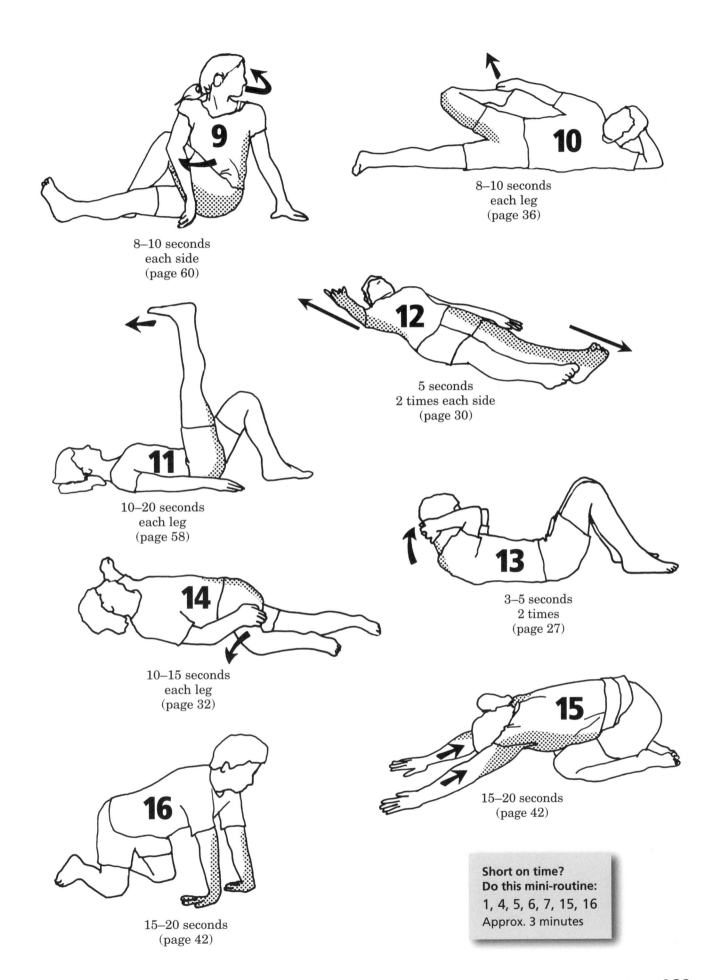

9

8–10 seconds
each side
(page 60)

10

8–10 seconds
each leg
(page 36)

12

5 seconds
2 times each side
(page 30)

11

10–20 seconds
each leg
(page 58)

13

3–5 seconds
2 times
(page 27)

14

10–15 seconds
each leg
(page 32)

15

15–20 seconds
(page 42)

16

15–20 seconds
(page 42)

Short on time?
Do this mini-routine:
1, 4, 5, 6, 7, 15, 16
Approx. 3 minutes

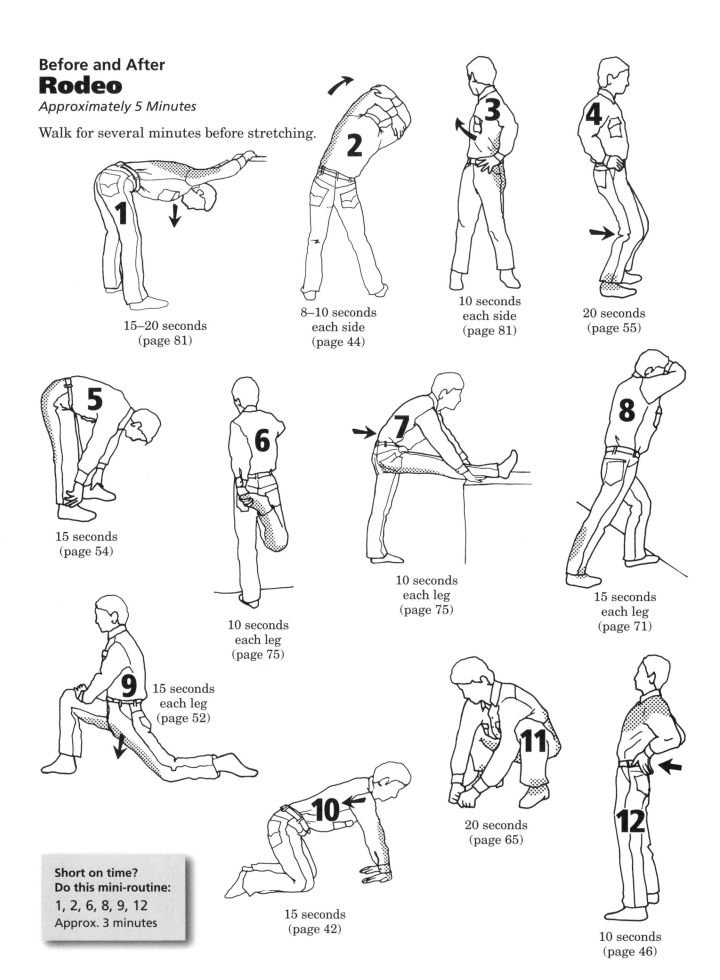

Before and After
Rodeo
Approximately 5 Minutes

Walk for several minutes before stretching.

1 15–20 seconds (page 81)

2 8–10 seconds each side (page 44)

3 10 seconds each side (page 81)

4 20 seconds (page 55)

5 15 seconds (page 54)

6 10 seconds each leg (page 75)

7 10 seconds each leg (page 75)

8 15 seconds each leg (page 71)

9 15 seconds each leg (page 52)

10 15 seconds (page 42)

11 20 seconds (page 65)

12 10 seconds (page 46)

Short on time?
Do this mini-routine:
1, 2, 6, 8, 9, 12
Approx. 3 minutes

Before and After
Rowing
Approximately 6 Minutes

Warm up by moving for 3–5 minutes before stretching.

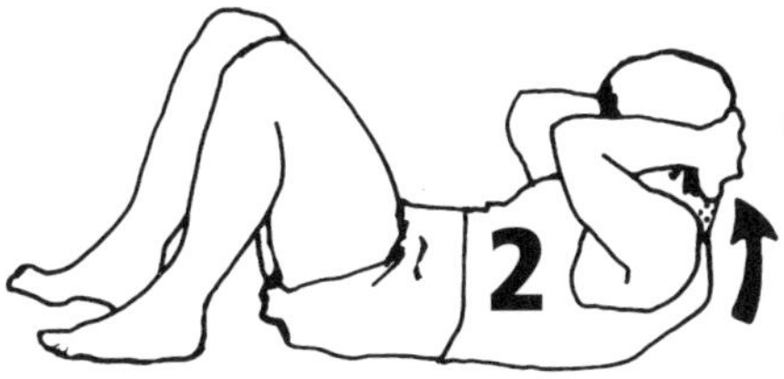

2 Contract 3–5 seconds then relax 2 times (page 27)

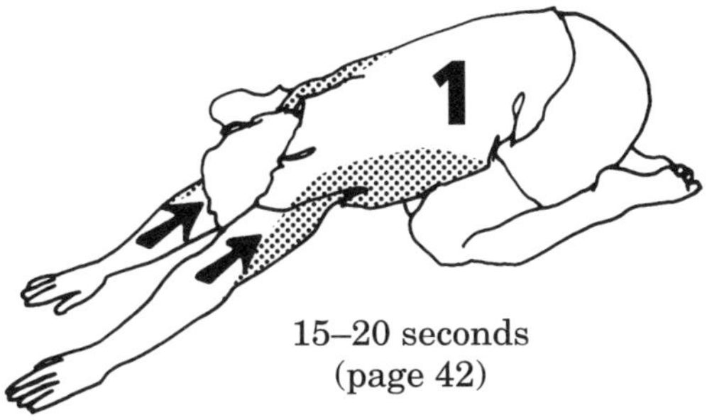

1 15–20 seconds (page 42)

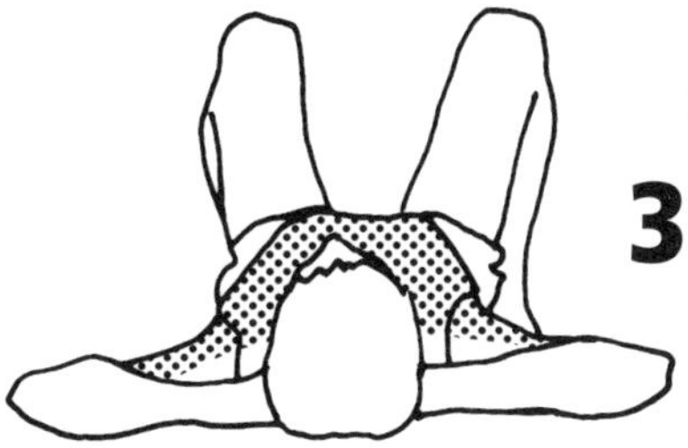

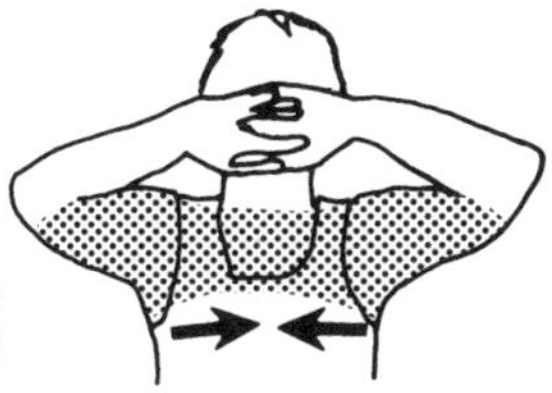

3 5 seconds 2 times (page 28)

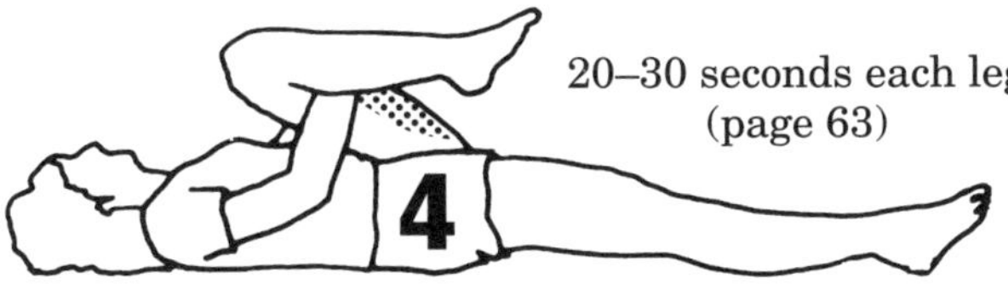

4 20–30 seconds each leg (page 63)

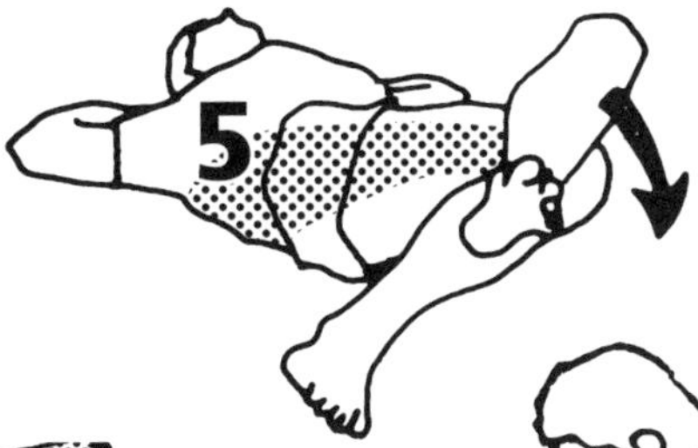

5 15–30 seconds each leg (page 27)

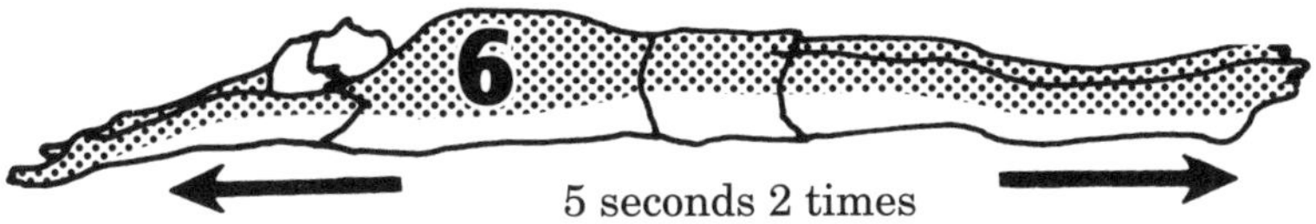

6 5 seconds 2 times (page 30)

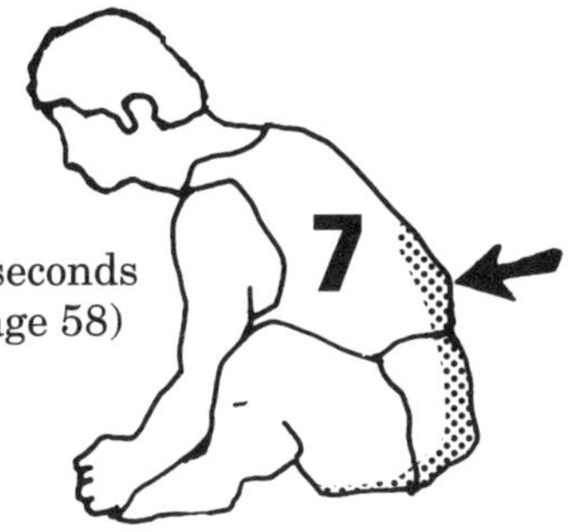

7 20 seconds (page 58)

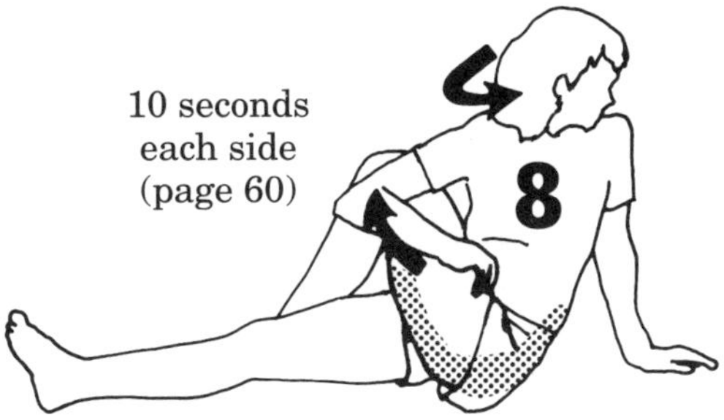

8 10 seconds each side (page 60)

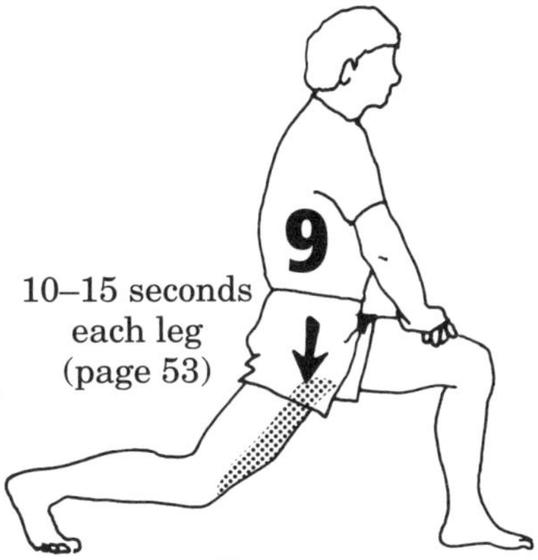

9 10–15 seconds each leg (page 53)

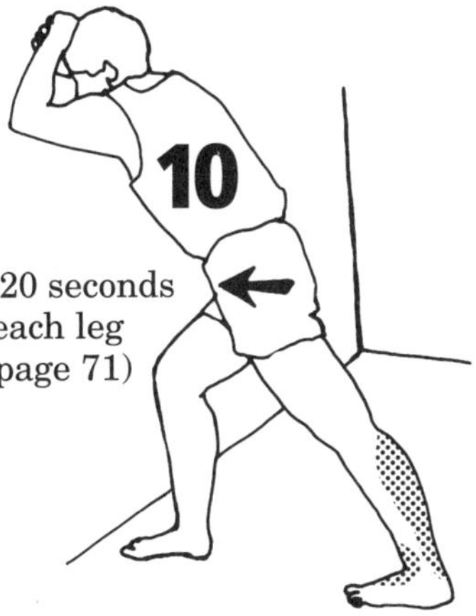

10 15–20 seconds each leg (page 71)

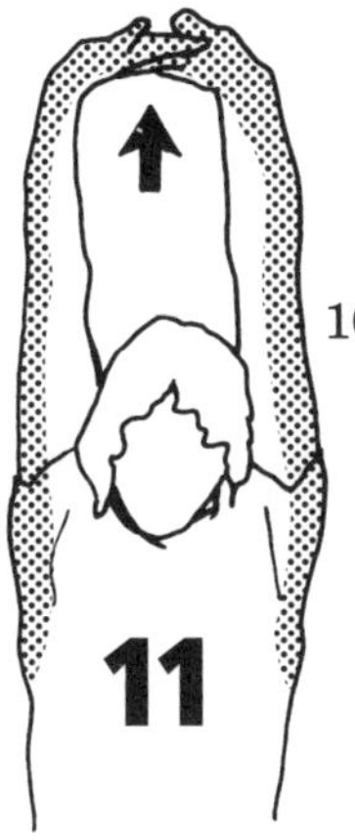

11 10–15 seconds (page 46)

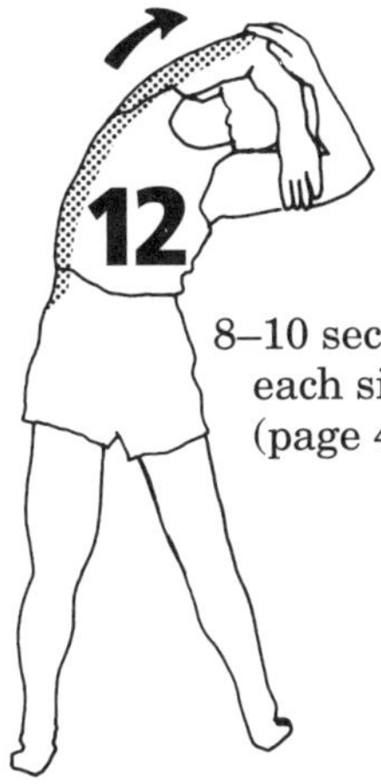

12 8–10 seconds each side (page 44)

Short on time?
Do this mini-routine:
1, 7, 9, 10, 11, 12
Approx. 3 minutes

Before
Running
Approximately 4 Minutes

Warm up by jogging for 3–5 minutes before stretching.

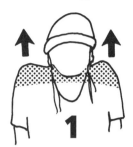

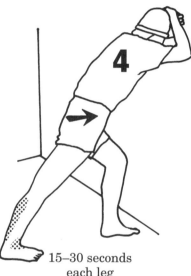

3–5 seconds
2 times
(page 46)

8–10 seconds
each side
(page 44)

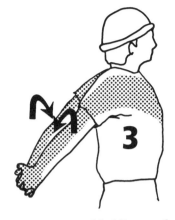

10–15 seconds
(page 47)

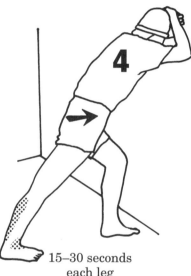

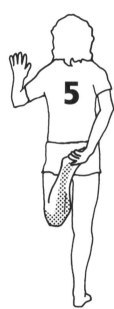

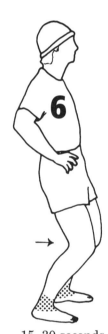

15–30 seconds
each leg
(page 71)

10–15 seconds
each leg
(page 75)

15–30 seconds
(page 55)

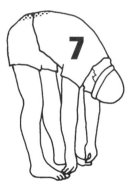

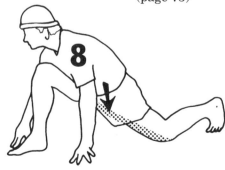

10–15 seconds
(page 54)

15 seconds
each leg
(page 51)

Short on time?
After a mild warm-up of 2–3 minutes, do this mini-routine:
3, 4, 5, 8
Approx. 1½ minutes

Stretching © 2000 by Bob and Jean Anderson. Shelter Publications, Inc.

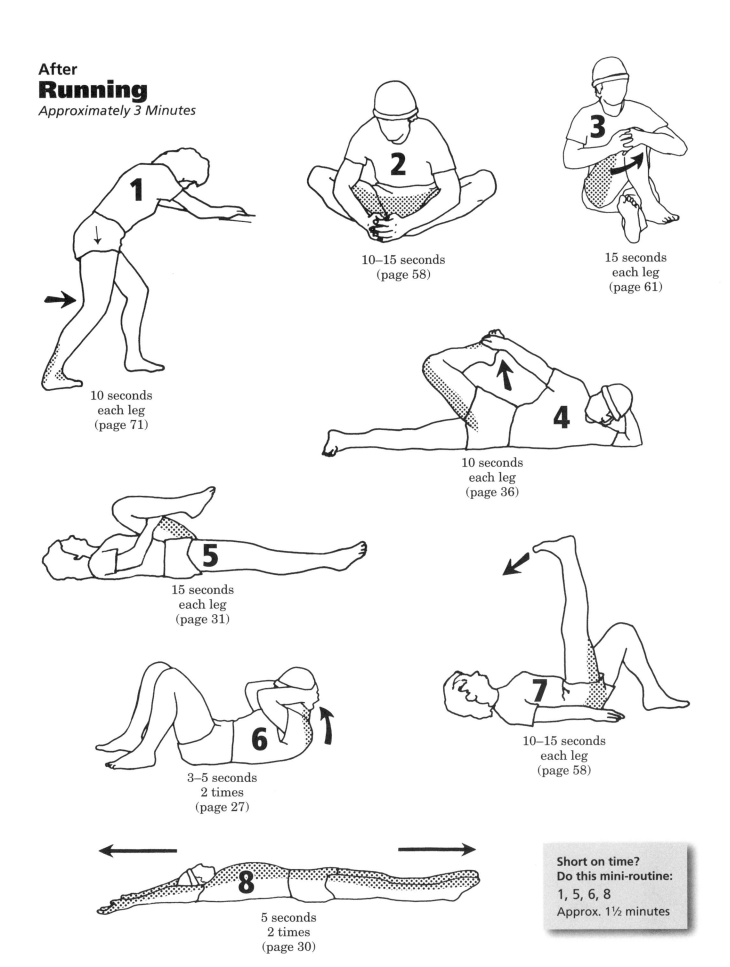

Running
Approximately 3 Minutes

1

10 seconds
each leg
(page 71)

2

10–15 seconds
(page 58)

3

15 seconds
each leg
(page 61)

4

10 seconds
each leg
(page 36)

5

15 seconds
each leg
(page 31)

6

3–5 seconds
2 times
(page 27)

7

10–15 seconds
each leg
(page 58)

8

5 seconds
2 times
(page 30)

Short on time?
Do this mini-routine:
1, 5, 6, 8
Approx. 1½ minutes

Stretching © 2000 by Bob and Jean Anderson. Shelter Publications, Inc.

Skiing (Cross-Country)

Approximately 3 Minutes

Warm up by walking for several minutes with a big arm swing before stretching.

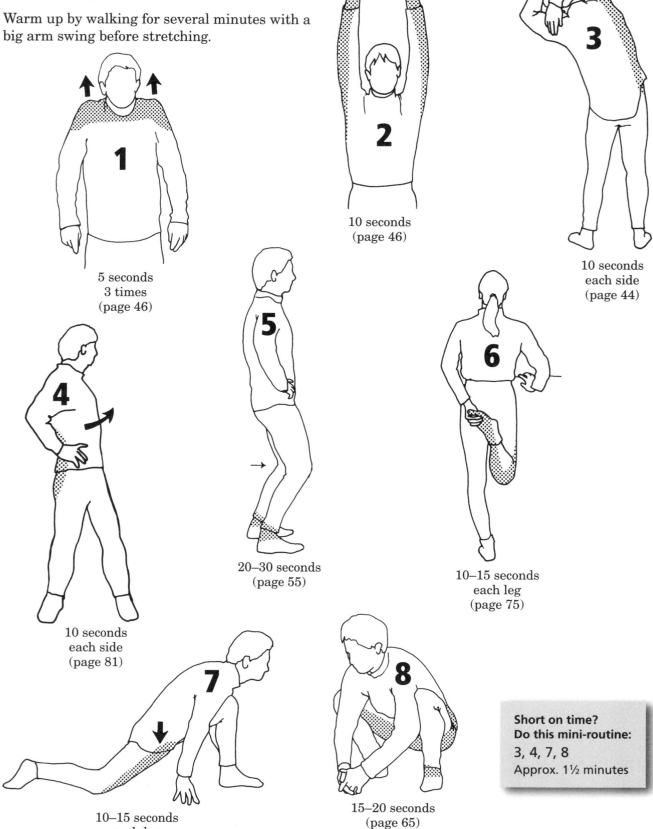

5 seconds
3 times
(page 46)

10 seconds
(page 46)

10 seconds
each side
(page 44)

10 seconds
each side
(page 81)

20–30 seconds
(page 55)

10–15 seconds
each leg
(page 75)

10–15 seconds
each leg
(page 51)

15–20 seconds
(page 65)

Short on time?
Do this mini-routine:
3, 4, 7, 8
Approx. 1½ minutes

1

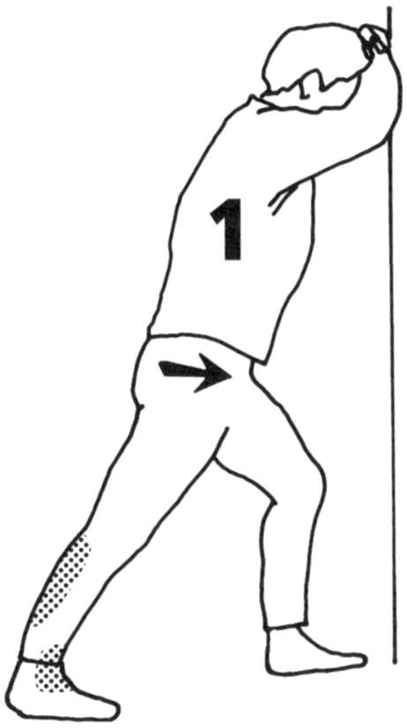

15–20 seconds
each leg
(page 71)

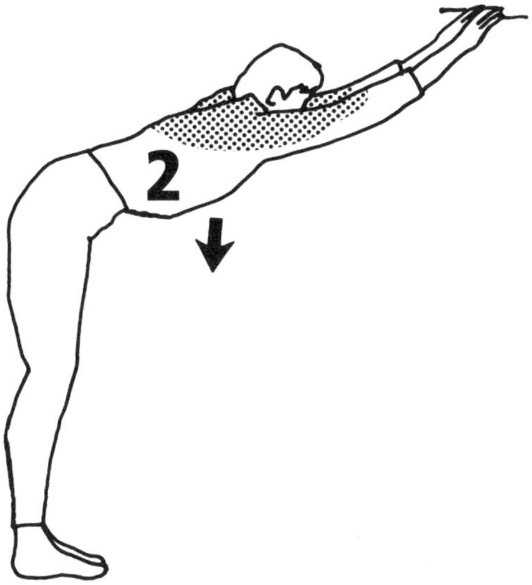

2

10–15 seconds
(page 81)

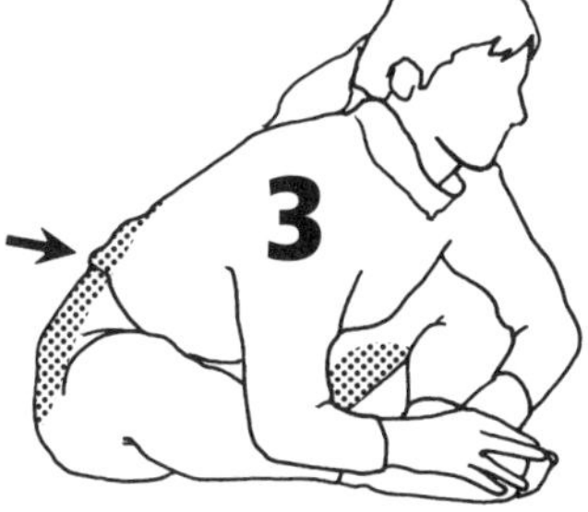

3

10–15 seconds
(page 58)

4

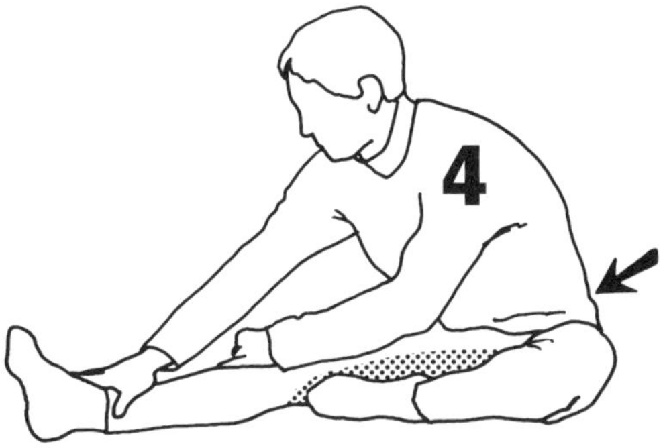

10–15 seconds
each leg
(page 39)

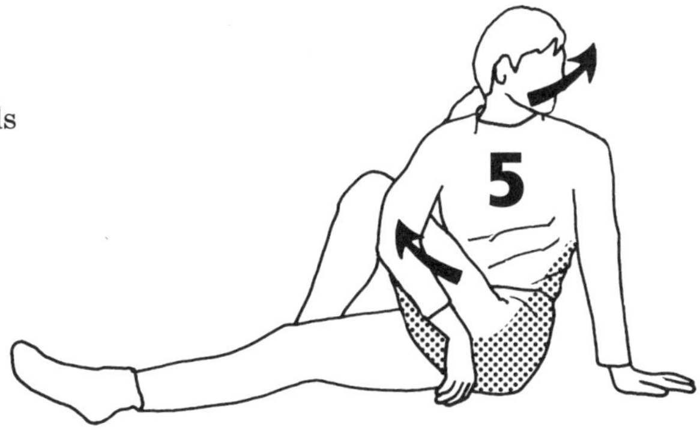

5

8–10 seconds
each side
(page 60)

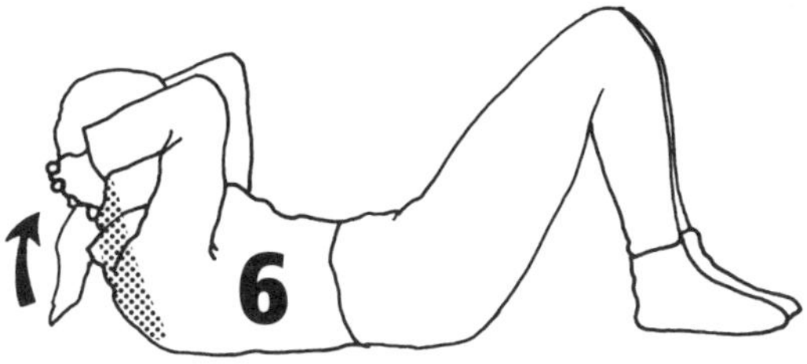

6

3–5 seconds
2 times
(page 27)

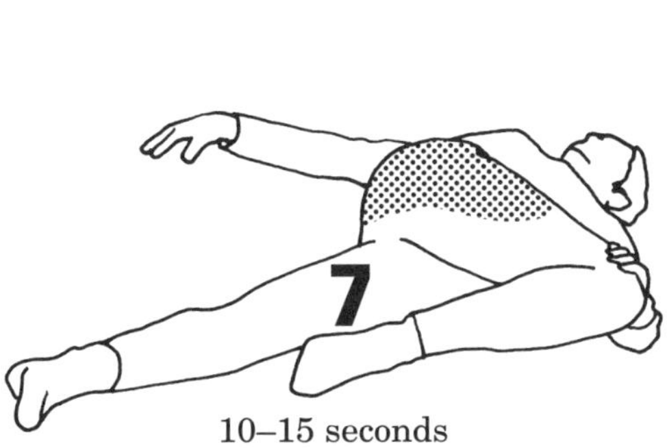

7

10–15 seconds
each side
(page 32)

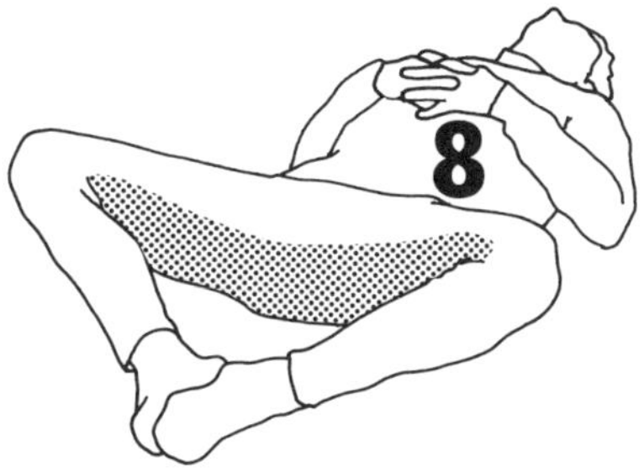

8

20–30 seconds
(page 26)

Short on time?
Do this mini-routine:
1, 3, 4, 5
Approx. 2 minutes

Before
Skiing (Downhill)
Approximately 3 Minutes

Walk for 2–3 minutes.

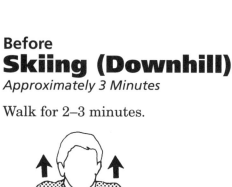

5 seconds
2 times
(page 46)

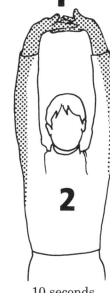

10 seconds
(page 46)

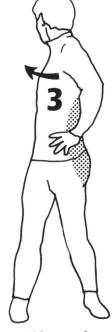

10 seconds
each side
(page 81)

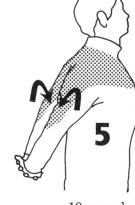

8–10 seconds
each side
(page 44)

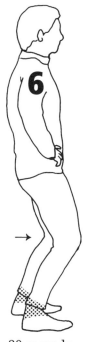

10 seconds
(page 47)

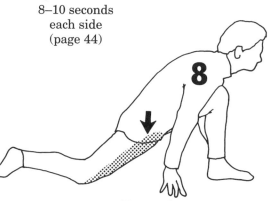

30 seconds
(page 55)

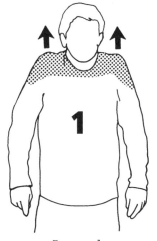

10–15 seconds
each leg
(page 75)

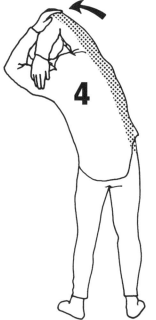

15 seconds
each leg
(page 51)

Short on time?
Do this mini-routine:
2, 3, 6, 8
Approx. 1½ minutes

Stretching © 2000 by Bob and Jean Anderson. Shelter Publications, Inc.

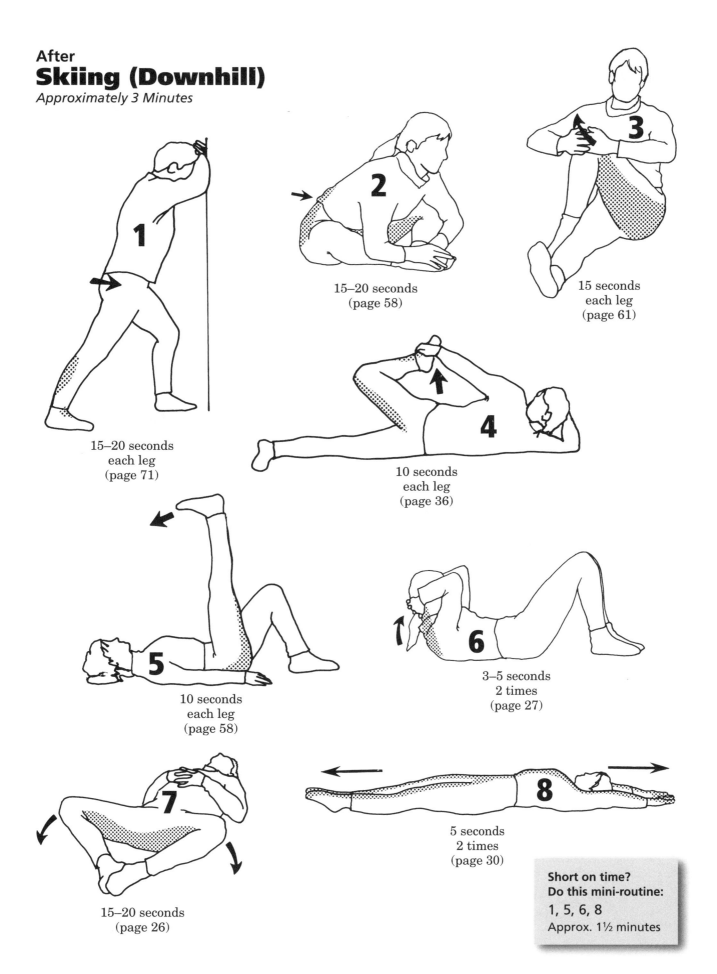

15–20 seconds
each leg
(page 71)

15–20 seconds
(page 58)

15 seconds
each leg
(page 61)

10 seconds
each leg
(page 36)

10 seconds
each leg
(page 58)

3–5 seconds
2 times
(page 27)

15–20 seconds
(page 26)

5 seconds
2 times
(page 30)

Short on time?
Do this mini-routine:
1, 5, 6, 8
Approx. 1½ minutes

Before and After
Snowboarding
Approximately 5 Minutes

Walk for several minutes before
stretching.

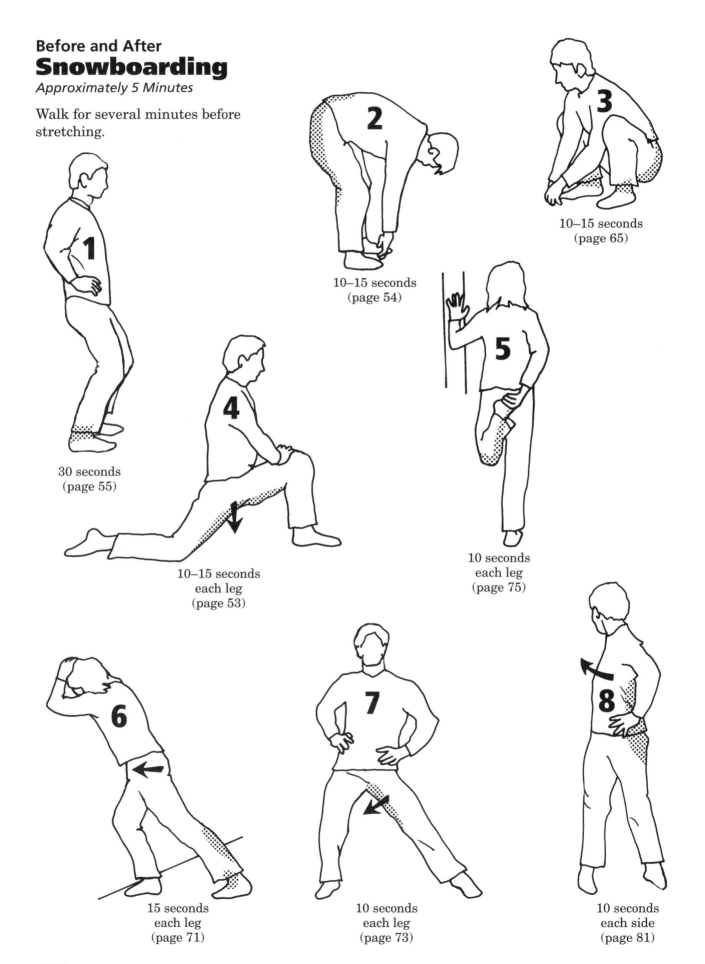

30 seconds
(page 55)

10–15 seconds
(page 54)

10–15 seconds
(page 65)

10–15 seconds
each leg
(page 53)

10 seconds
each leg
(page 75)

15 seconds
each leg
(page 71)

10 seconds
each leg
(page 73)

10 seconds
each side
(page 81)

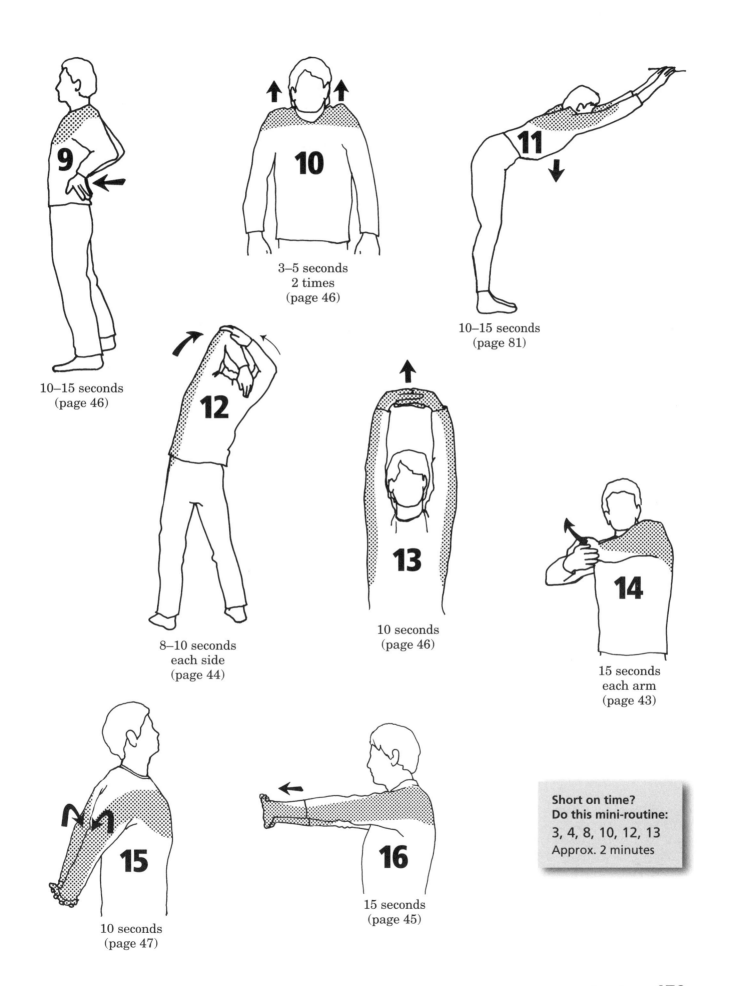

9

10–15 seconds
(page 46)

10

3–5 seconds
2 times
(page 46)

11

10–15 seconds
(page 81)

12

8–10 seconds
each side
(page 44)

13

10 seconds
(page 46)

14

15 seconds
each arm
(page 43)

15

10 seconds
(page 47)

16

15 seconds
(page 45)

Short on time?
Do this mini-routine:
3, 4, 8, 10, 12, 13
Approx. 2 minutes

Before
Soccer

Approximately 3 Minutes

Jog around the soccer field before stretching.

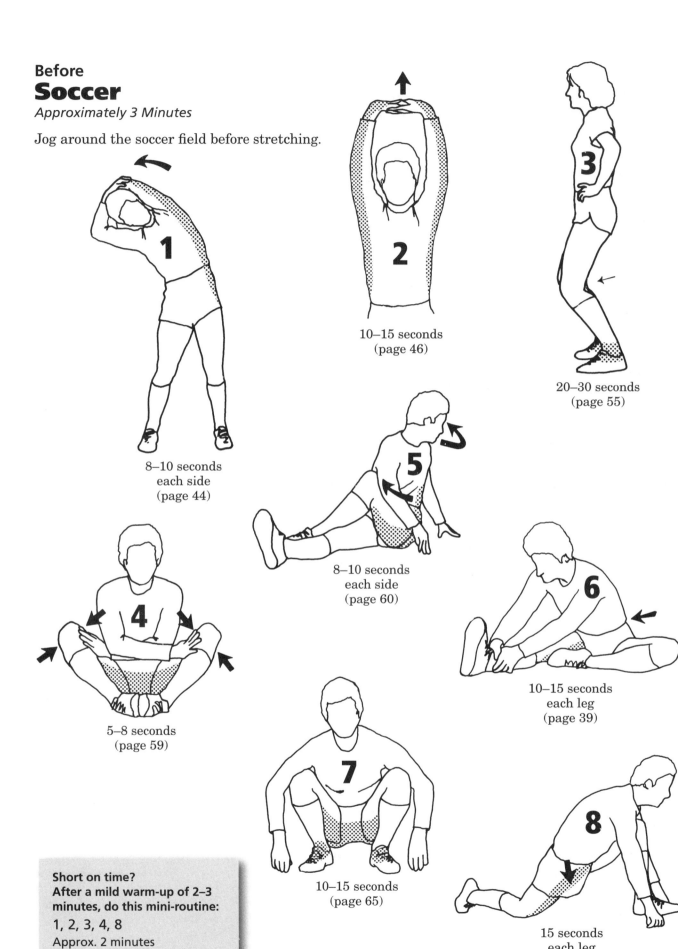

1
8–10 seconds
each side
(page 44)

2
10–15 seconds
(page 46)

3
20–30 seconds
(page 55)

4
5–8 seconds
(page 59)

5
8–10 seconds
each side
(page 60)

6
10–15 seconds
each leg
(page 39)

7
10–15 seconds
(page 65)

8
15 seconds
each leg
(page 52)

Short on time?
After a mild warm-up of 2–3
minutes, do this mini-routine:

1, 2, 3, 4, 8
Approx. 2 minutes

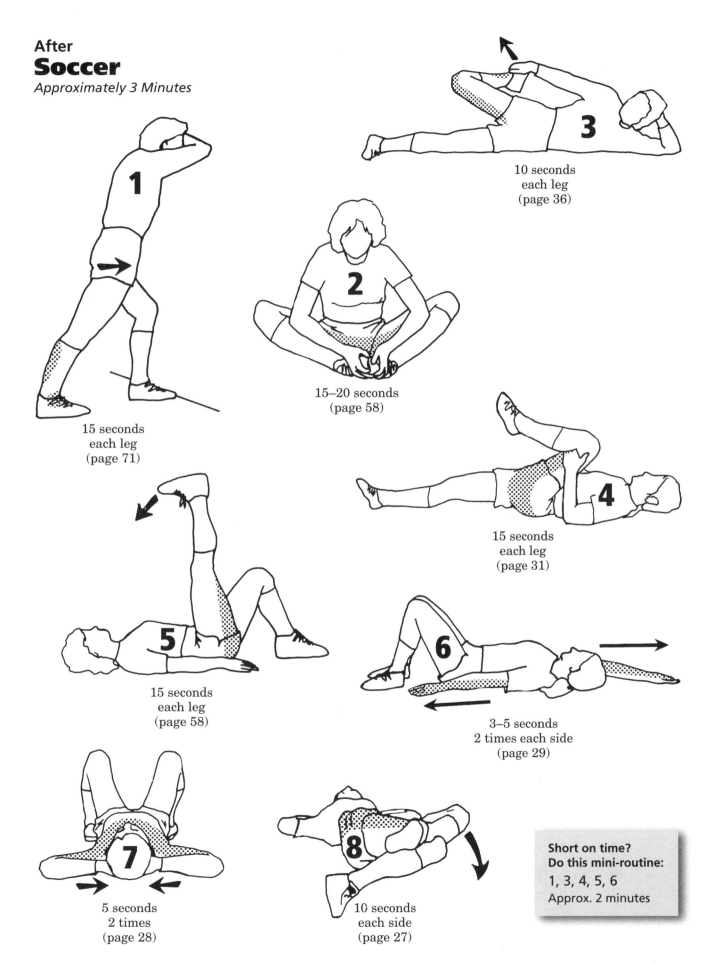

After
Soccer
Approximately 3 Minutes

1

15 seconds
each leg
(page 71)

2

15–20 seconds
(page 58)

3

10 seconds
each leg
(page 36)

4

15 seconds
each leg
(page 31)

5

15 seconds
each leg
(page 58)

6

3–5 seconds
2 times each side
(page 29)

7

5 seconds
2 times
(page 28)

8

10 seconds
each side
(page 27)

Short on time?
Do this mini-routine:
1, 3, 4, 5, 6
Approx. 2 minutes

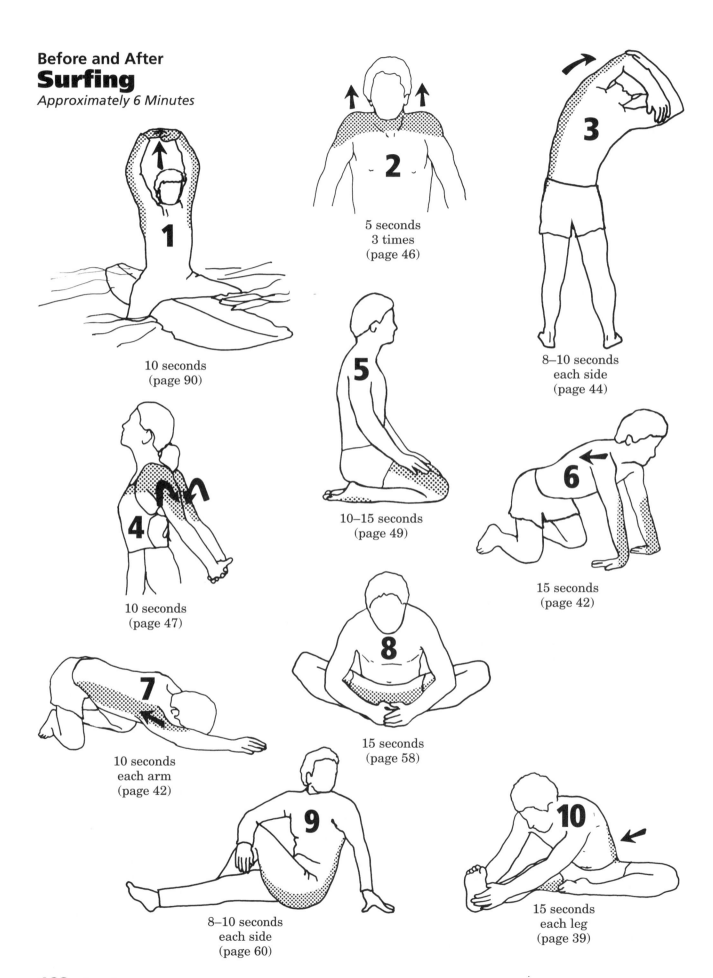

Before and After
Surfing
Approximately 6 Minutes

1

10 seconds
(page 90)

2

5 seconds
3 times
(page 46)

3

8–10 seconds
each side
(page 44)

4

10 seconds
(page 47)

5

10–15 seconds
(page 49)

6

15 seconds
(page 42)

7

10 seconds
each arm
(page 42)

8

15 seconds
(page 58)

9

8–10 seconds
each side
(page 60)

10

15 seconds
each leg
(page 39)

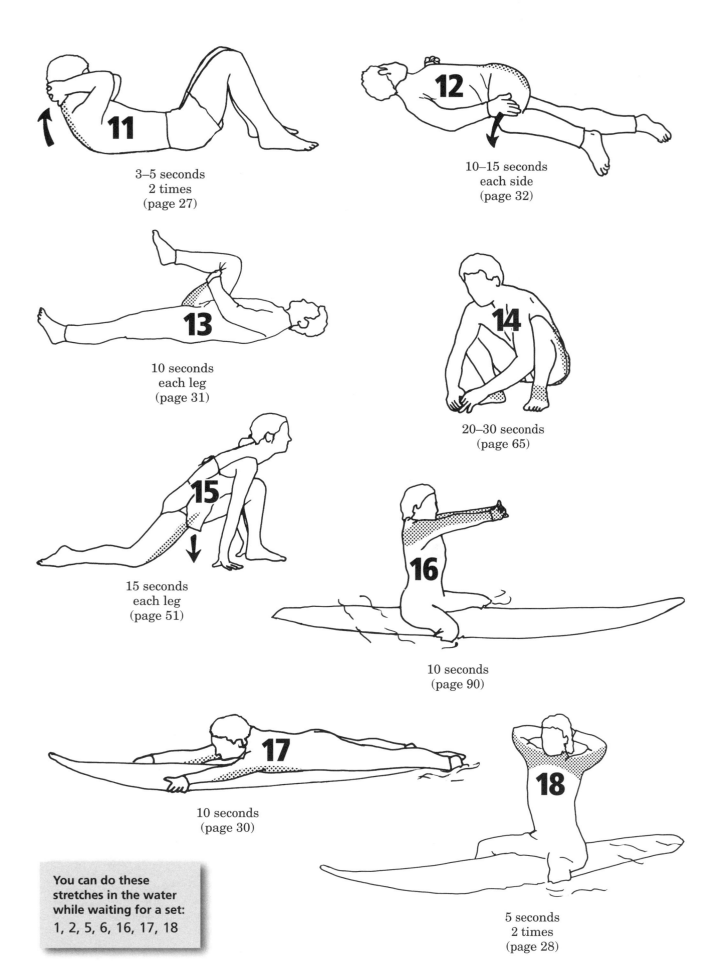

11
3–5 seconds
2 times
(page 27)

12
10–15 seconds
each side
(page 32)

13
10 seconds
each leg
(page 31)

14
20–30 seconds
(page 65)

15
15 seconds
each leg
(page 51)

16
10 seconds
(page 90)

17
10 seconds
(page 30)

18
5 seconds
2 times
(page 28)

**You can do these
stretches in the water
while waiting for a set:**
1, 2, 5, 6, 16, 17, 18

Before and After
Swimming
Approximately 5 Minutes

Walk with a big arm swing for 2–3 minutes before stretching.

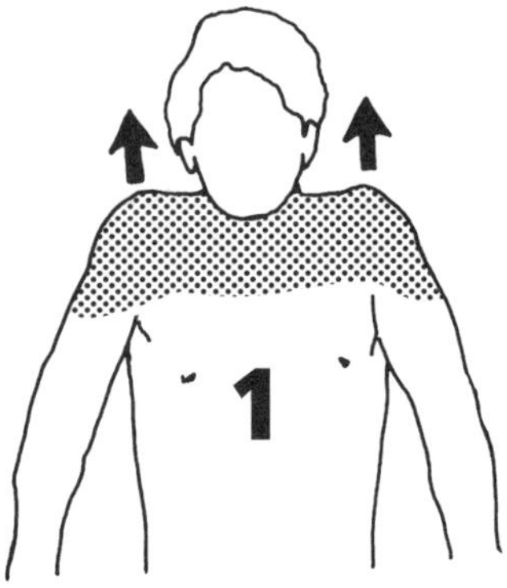

5 seconds
3 times
(page 46)

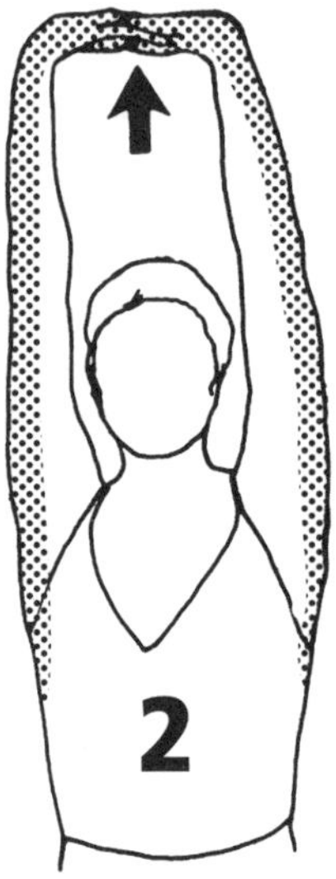

10–15 seconds
(page 46)

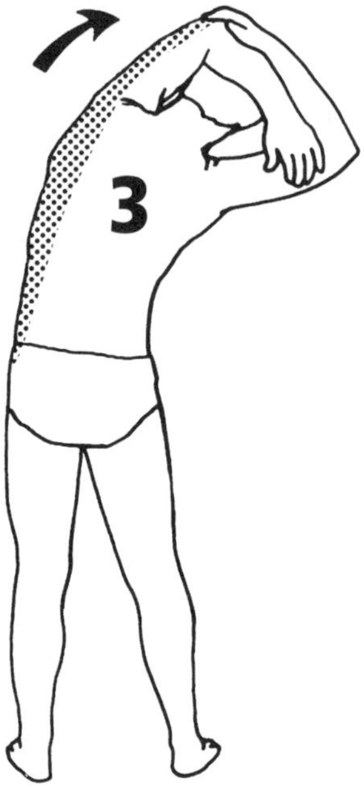

10 seconds
each side
(page 44)

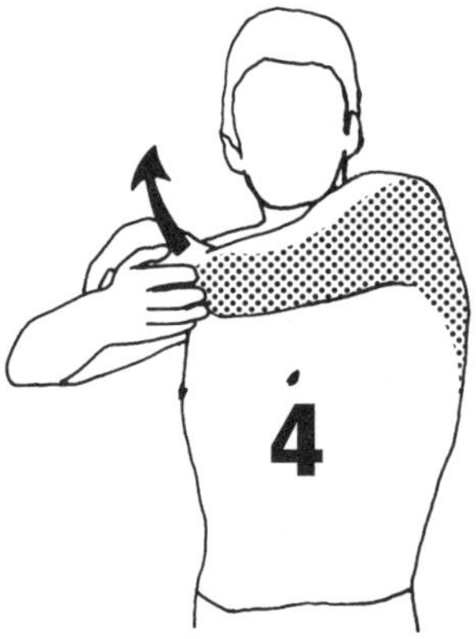

15 seconds
each arm
(page 43)

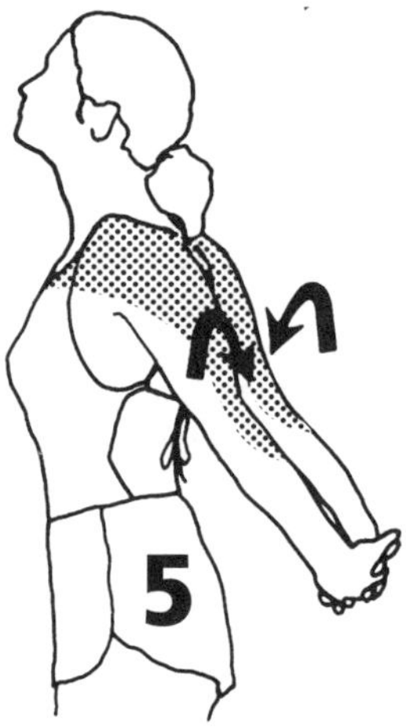

15 seconds
(page 47)

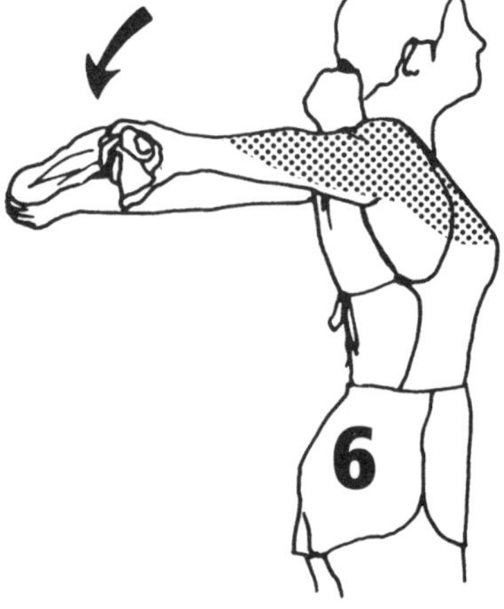

10 seconds
(page 87)

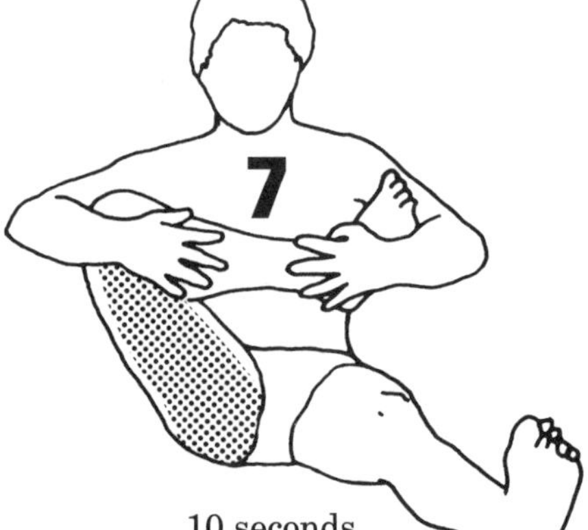

10 seconds
each leg
(page 35)

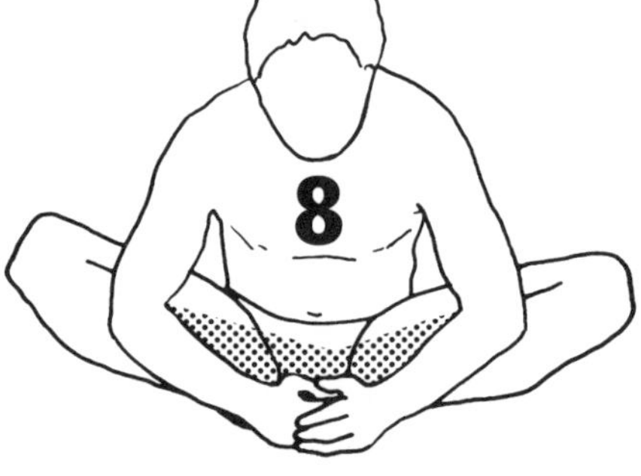

15 seconds
(page 58)

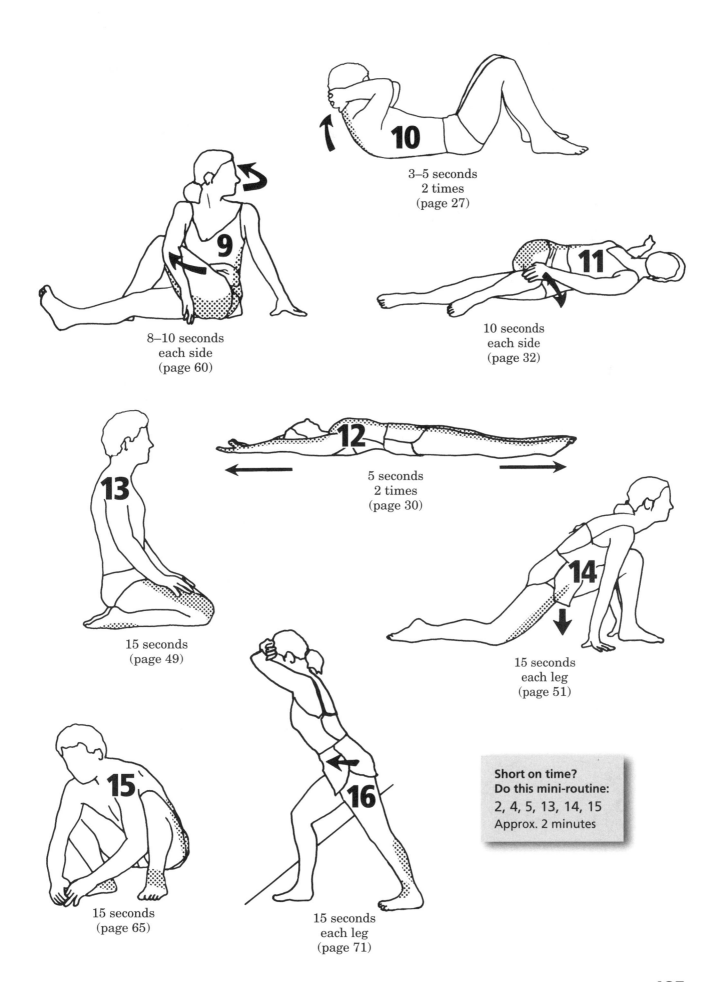

9
8–10 seconds
each side
(page 60)

10
3–5 seconds
2 times
(page 27)

11
10 seconds
each side
(page 32)

12
5 seconds
2 times
(page 30)

13
15 seconds
(page 49)

14
15 seconds
each leg
(page 51)

15
15 seconds
(page 65)

16
15 seconds
each leg
(page 71)

Short on time?
Do this mini-routine:
2, 4, 5, 13, 14, 15
Approx. 2 minutes

Before and After
Table Tennis
Approximately 5 Minutes

Walk for several minutes before stretching.

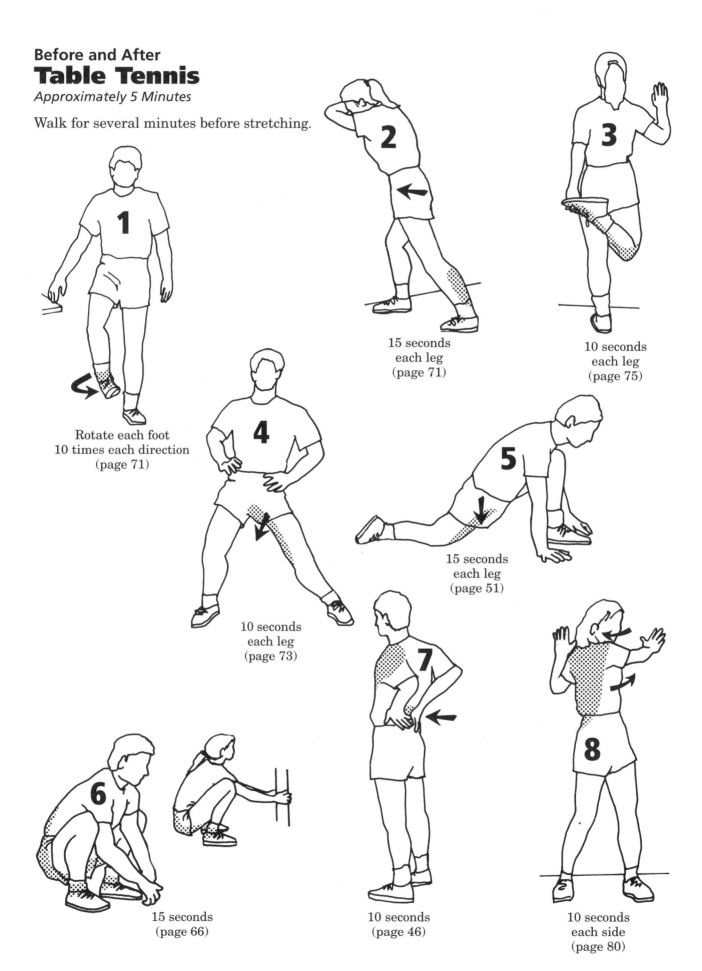

Rotate each foot
10 times each direction
(page 71)

15 seconds
each leg
(page 71)

10 seconds
each leg
(page 75)

10 seconds
each leg
(page 73)

15 seconds
each leg
(page 51)

15 seconds
(page 66)

10 seconds
(page 46)

10 seconds
each side
(page 80)

Stretching © 2000 by Bob and Jean Anderson. Shelter Publications, Inc.

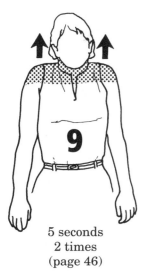

5 seconds
2 times
(page 46)

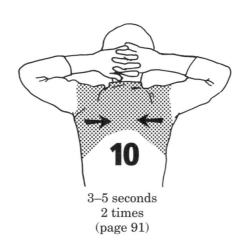

3–5 seconds
2 times
(page 91)

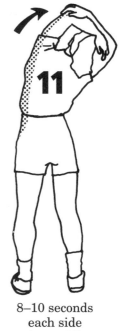

8–10 seconds
each side
(page 44)

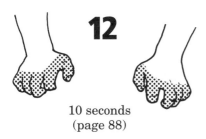

10 seconds
(page 88)

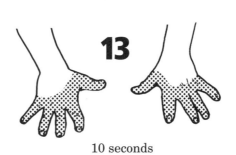

10 seconds
(page 88)

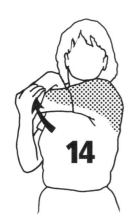

15 seconds
each arm
(page 43)

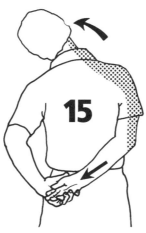

10 seconds
each arm
(page 47)

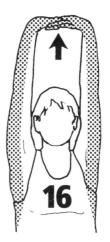

15 seconds
(page 46)

Short on time?
Do this mini-routine:
2, 3, 5, 8, 10, 11, 15
Approx. 1½ minutes

Before and After
Tennis
Approximately 5 Minutes

Walk or jog for several minutes before stretching.

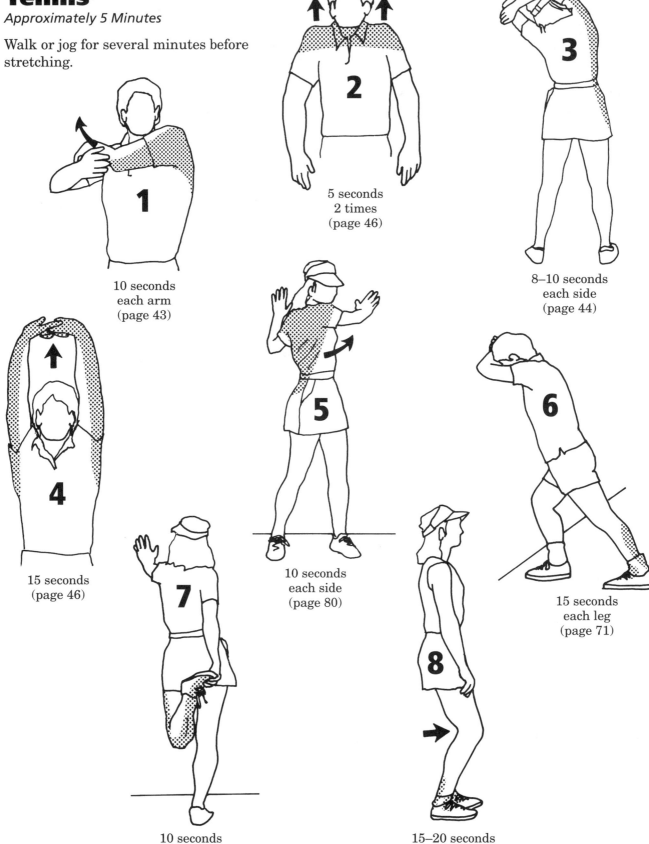

10 seconds
each arm
(page 43)

5 seconds
2 times
(page 46)

8–10 seconds
each side
(page 44)

15 seconds
(page 46)

10 seconds
each side
(page 80)

15 seconds
each leg
(page 71)

10 seconds
each leg
(page 75)

15–20 seconds
(page 55)

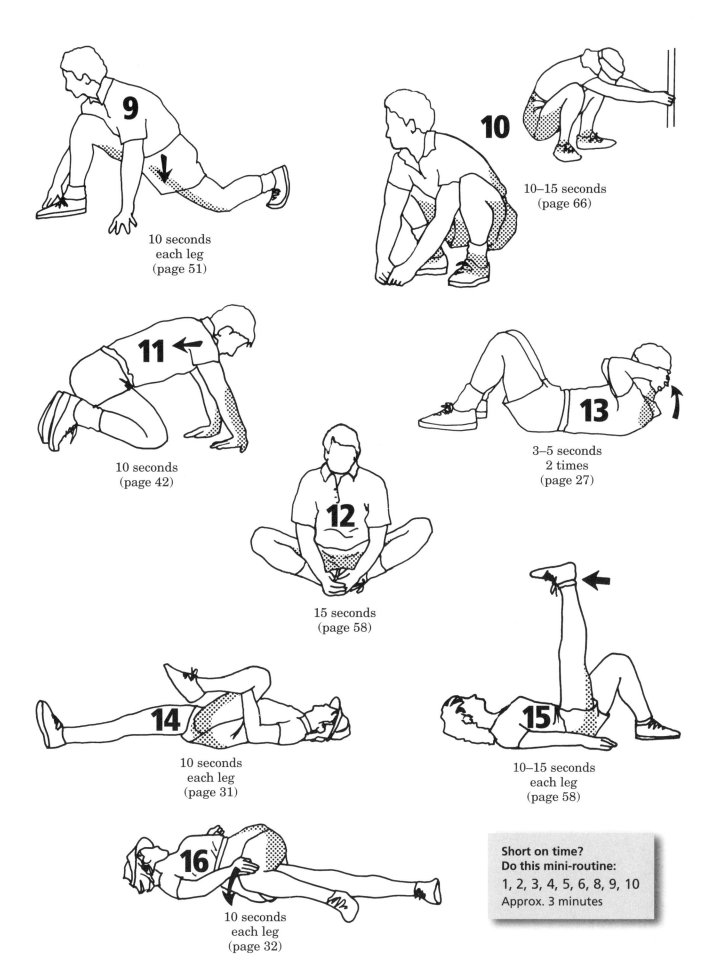

9

10 seconds
each leg
(page 51)

10

10–15 seconds
(page 66)

11

10 seconds
(page 42)

12

15 seconds
(page 58)

13

3–5 seconds
2 times
(page 27)

14

10 seconds
each leg
(page 31)

15

10–15 seconds
each leg
(page 58)

16

10 seconds
each leg
(page 32)

Short on time?
Do this mini-routine:
1, 2, 3, 4, 5, 6, 8, 9, 10
Approx. 3 minutes

Before and After
Triathlon (Swimming)
Approximately 2½ Minutes

Walk for several minutes before stretching.

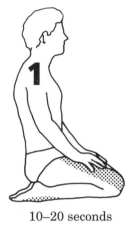

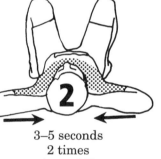

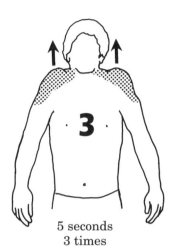

10–20 seconds
(page 49)

10–15 seconds
each arm
(page 42)

5 seconds
3 times
(page 46)

Before and After
Triathlon (Cycling)
Approximately 2 Minutes

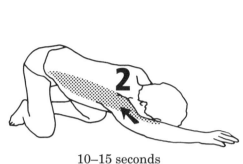

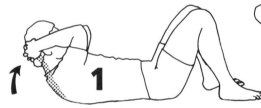

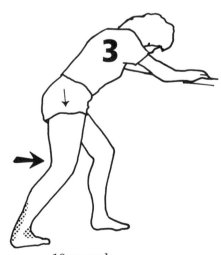

3–5 seconds
2 times
(page 28)

3–5 seconds
2 times
(page 27)

20–30 seconds
(page 26)

Before and After
Triathlon (Running)
Approximately 2 Minutes

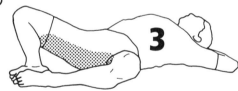

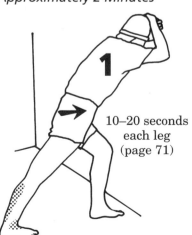

10–20 seconds
each leg
(page 71)

10–15 seconds
each leg
(page 75)

10 seconds
each leg
(page 71)

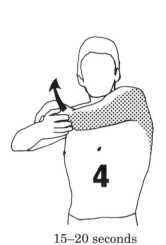

15–20 seconds
each arm
(page 43)

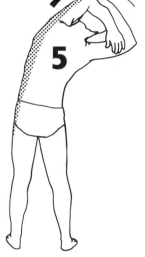

8–10 seconds
each side
(page 44)

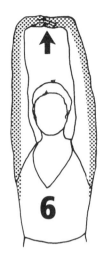

15–20 seconds
(page 46)

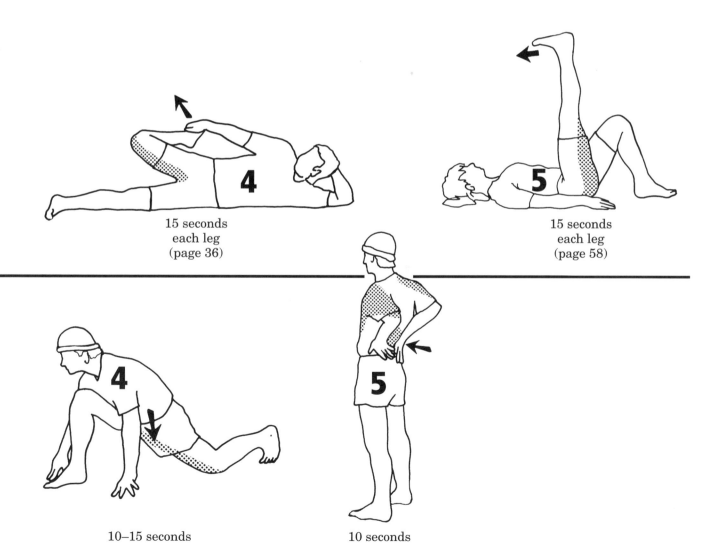

15 seconds
each leg
(page 36)

15 seconds
each leg
(page 58)

10–15 seconds
each leg
(page 51)

10 seconds
(page 46)

Before and After
Volleyball
Approximately 6 Minutes

Walk or jog for 2–3 minutes before stretching.

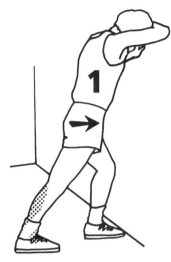

10–15 seconds
each leg
(page 71)

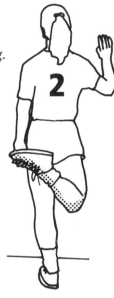

10 seconds
each leg
(page 75)

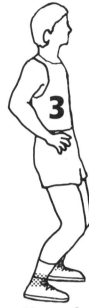

30 seconds
(page 55)

10–15 seconds
(page 54)

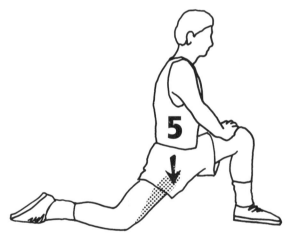

10–15 seconds
each leg
(page 53)

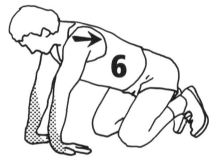

10–15 seconds
(page 42)

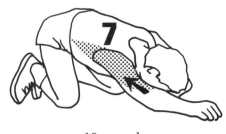

10 seconds
each arm
(page 42)

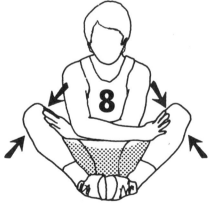

5–8 seconds
(page 59)

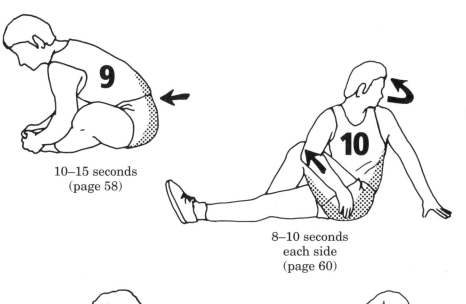

10–15 seconds
(page 58)

8–10 seconds
each side
(page 60)

20 seconds
(page 66)

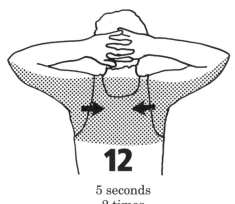

5 seconds
2 times
(page 91)

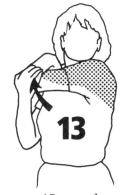

15 seconds
each arm
(page 43)

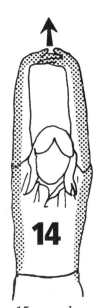

15 seconds
(page 46)

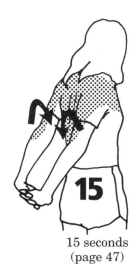

15 seconds
(page 47)

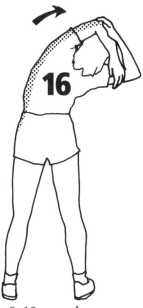

8–10 seconds
each side
(page 44)

Short on time?
Do this mini-routine:
1, 2, 3, 5, 13, 14, 15, 16
Approx. 3 minutes

Before and After
Weight Training
Approximately 7 Minutes

Warm up by using a stationary bike or treadmill, etc., for 3–5 minutes before stretching.

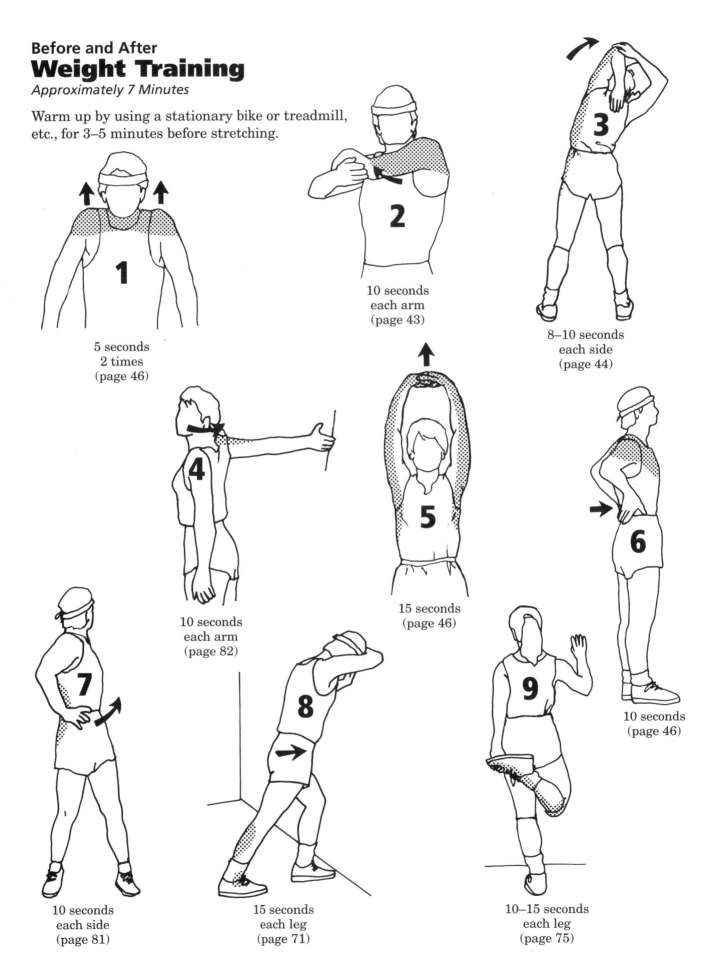

1
5 seconds
2 times
(page 46)

2
10 seconds
each arm
(page 43)

3
8–10 seconds
each side
(page 44)

4
10 seconds
each arm
(page 82)

5
15 seconds
(page 46)

6
10 seconds
(page 46)

7
10 seconds
each side
(page 81)

8
15 seconds
each leg
(page 71)

9
10–15 seconds
each leg
(page 75)

Stretching © 2000 by Bob and Jean Anderson. Shelter Publications, Inc.

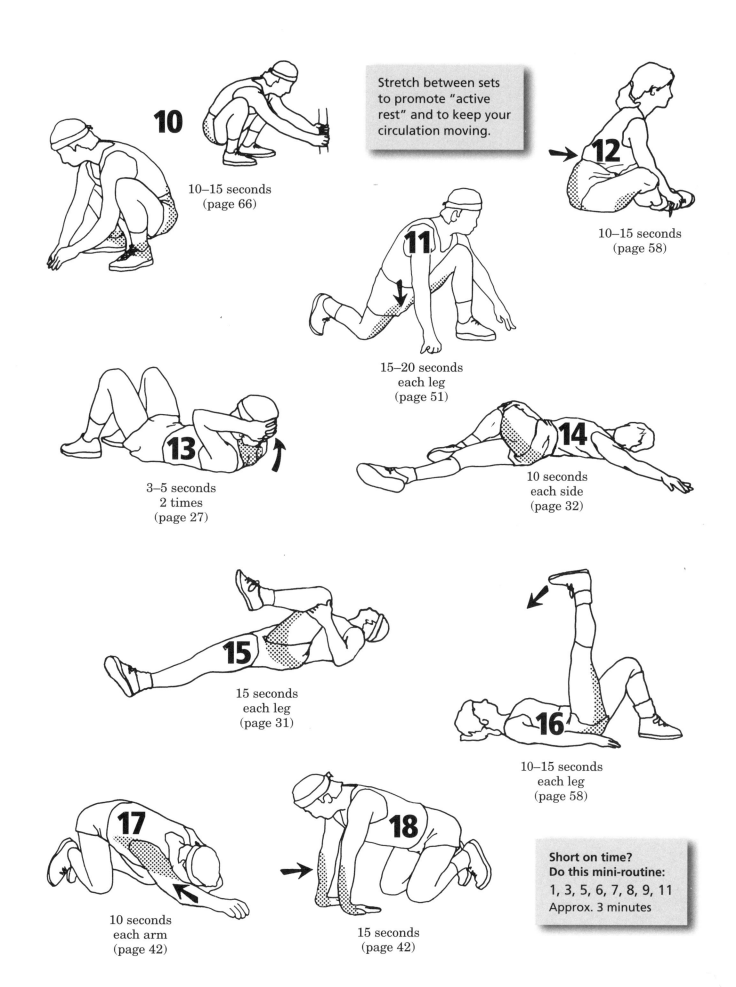

10

10–15 seconds
(page 66)

Stretch between sets
to promote "active
rest" and to keep your
circulation moving.

11

15–20 seconds
each leg
(page 51)

12

10–15 seconds
(page 58)

13

3–5 seconds
2 times
(page 27)

14

10 seconds
each side
(page 32)

15

15 seconds
each leg
(page 31)

16

10–15 seconds
each leg
(page 58)

17

10 seconds
each arm
(page 42)

18

15 seconds
(page 42)

Short on time?
Do this mini-routine:
1, 3, 5, 6, 7, 8, 9, 11
Approx. 3 minutes

Before and After
Windsurfing
Approximately 6 Minutes

Walk for several minutes before stretching.

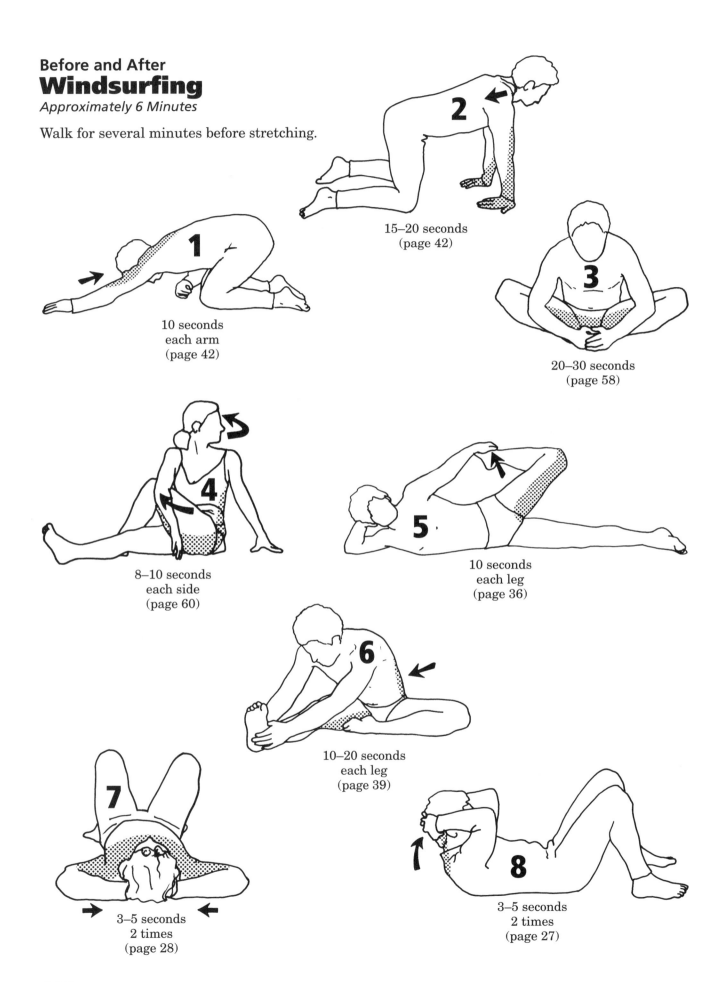

15–20 seconds
(page 42)

10 seconds
each arm
(page 42)

20–30 seconds
(page 58)

8–10 seconds
each side
(page 60)

10 seconds
each leg
(page 36)

10–20 seconds
each leg
(page 39)

3–5 seconds
2 times
(page 28)

3–5 seconds
2 times
(page 27)

Stretching © 2000 by Bob and Jean Anderson. Shelter Publications, Inc.

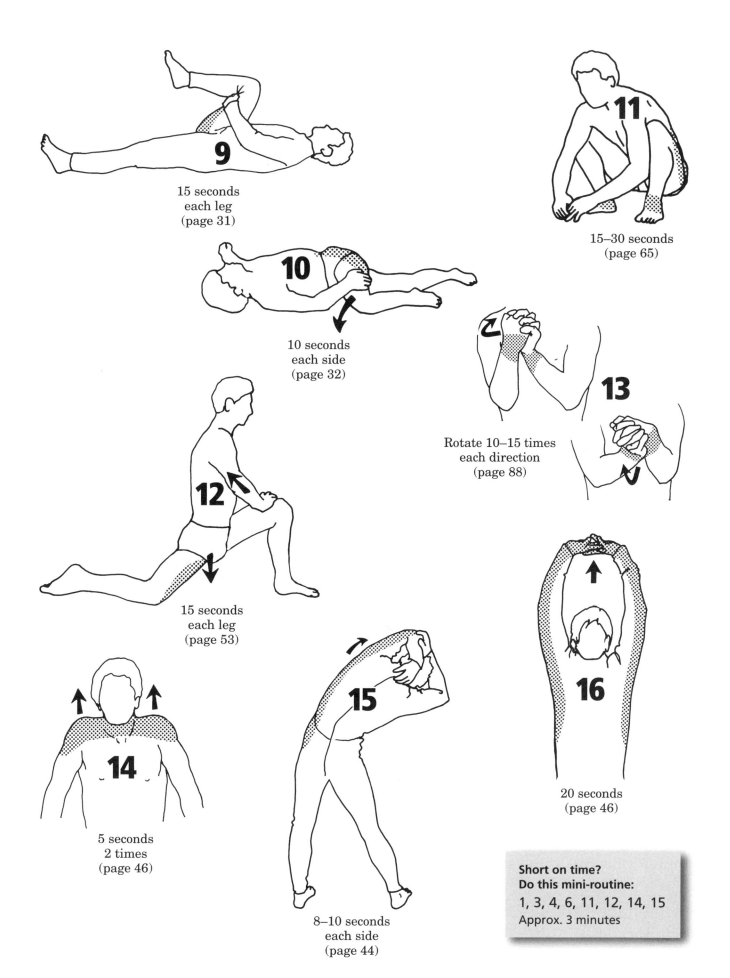

9
15 seconds
each leg
(page 31)

11
15–30 seconds
(page 65)

10
10 seconds
each side
(page 32)

13
Rotate 10–15 times
each direction
(page 88)

12
15 seconds
each leg
(page 53)

16
20 seconds
(page 46)

14
5 seconds
2 times
(page 46)

15
8–10 seconds
each side
(page 44)

Short on time?
Do this mini-routine:
1, 3, 4, 6, 11, 12, 14, 15
Approx. 3 minutes

Before and After
Wrestling
Approximately 6 Minutes

Jog for 2–3 minutes before stretching.

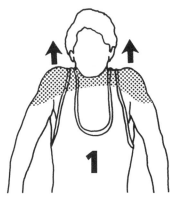

1

5 seconds
3 times
(page 46)

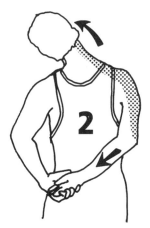

2

10 seconds
each arm
(page 47)

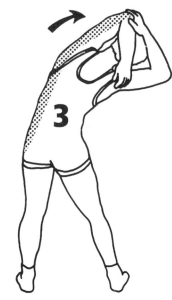

3

8–10 seconds
each side
(page 44)

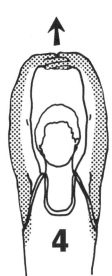

4

15 seconds
(page 46)

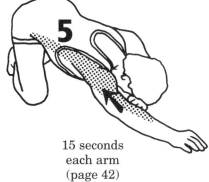

5

15 seconds
each arm
(page 42)

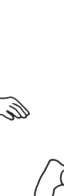

6

20 seconds
(page 42)

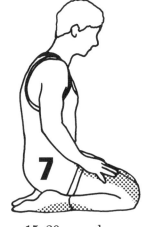

7

15–20 seconds
(page 49)

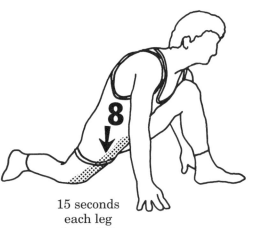

8

15 seconds
each leg
(page 51)

Stretching © 2000 by Bob and Jean Anderson. Shelter Publications, Inc.

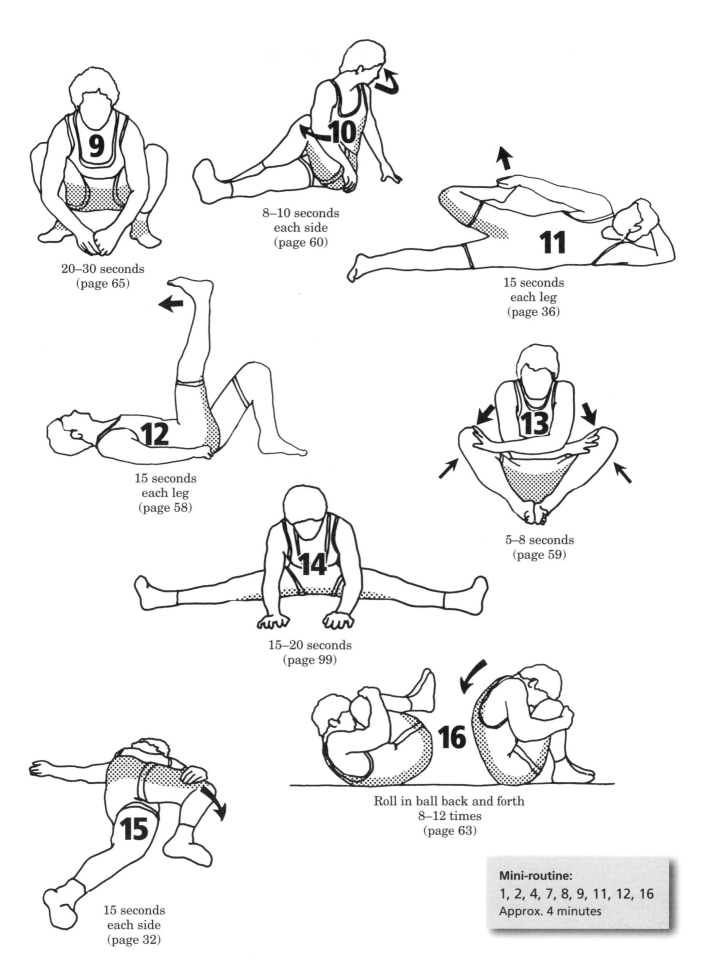

9
20–30 seconds
(page 65)

10
8–10 seconds
each side
(page 60)

11
15 seconds
each leg
(page 36)

12
15 seconds
each leg
(page 58)

13
5–8 seconds
(page 59)

14
15–20 seconds
(page 99)

16
Roll in ball back and forth
8–12 times
(page 63)

15
15 seconds
each side
(page 32)

Mini-routine:
1, 2, 4, 7, 8, 9, 11, 12, 16
Approx. 4 minutes

To Teachers and Coaches

For student athletes training has always stressed discipline, constantly pushing to new limits, and building maximum strength and power. As teachers and coaches, you are interested, of course, in team performance. But your most important goal is to educate the individuals under your supervision.

The best way to teach stretching is by your own example. When you yourself do the stretches and enjoy them, you will communicate this with enthusiasm. You will generate the same kind of attitude in your students.

In recent years, some attention has been given to stretching for injury prevention, but even here, there has been too much emphasis on maximum flexibility. *Stretching is entirely individual*. Let your students know that it is not a contest. There should be no comparisons made between students, because each is different. The emphasis should be on the feeling of the stretch, not on how far one can go. Stressing flexibility at the beginning will only lead to overstretching, a negative attitude, and possible injuries. If you notice someone who is tight or inflexible, don't single that person out; emphasize the proper stretches for that person alone, away from the group.

As a teacher/coach/guide, emphasize that stretching should be done with care and common sense. You do not have to set standards or push limits. Do not overwork or force your students to do too much. They will soon discover what feels right to them. They will improve naturally—and enjoy it.

It is important for students to understand that each and every one of them is an individual, with his or her own limits and a certain potential. All they can do is their best, nothing more.

The greatest gift you can give your students is to prepare them for the future. Teach them the value of regular exercise, of stretching daily, and of eating sensibly. Impress upon them that everyone can be fit, regardless of strength or athletic ability. Instill in your students an enthusiasm for movement and health that will last a lifetime.

APPENDIX

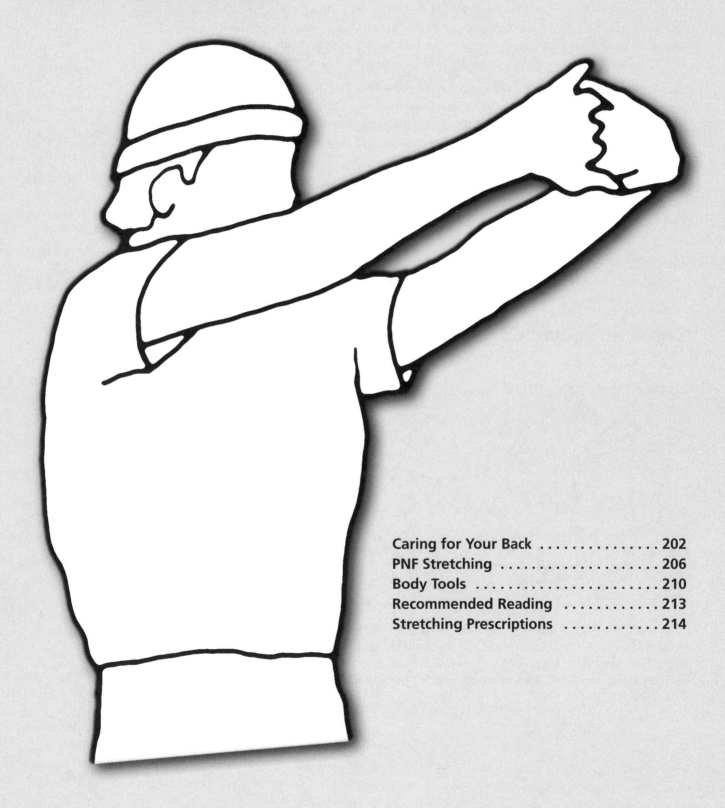

Caring for Your Back

More than 50 percent of all Americans will suffer from some sort of back problem some time during their lives. Some problems may be congenital, such as sway back or *scoliosis* (lateral curvature of the spine). Others may be the result of an automobile accident, a fall, or sports injury (in which case the pain may subside, only to reappear years later). But most back problems are simply due to tension and muscular tightness, which come from poor posture, being overweight, inactivity, and lack of abdominal strength.

Stretching and abdominal exercises can help your back if done with common sense. If you have a back problem, consult a reliable physician who will give you tests to see exactly where the problem lies. Ask your physician which of the stretches and exercises shown in this book would be of most help to you.

Anyone with a history of lower back problems should avoid stretches, called hyperextensions, that arch the back. They create too much stress on the lower back, and for this reason I have not included any such stretches in this book.

The best way to take care of your back is to use proper methods of stretching, strengthening, standing, sitting, and sleeping. For it is what we do moment to moment, day to day, that determines our total health. In the following pages are some suggestions for back care. *(Also see pp. 26–33.)*

Some Suggestions for Back Care and Posture

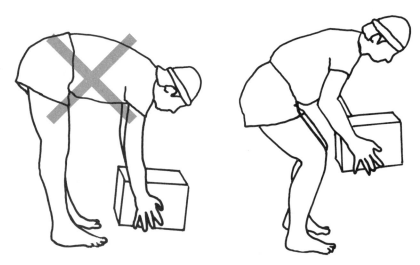

Never lift anything (heavy *or* light) with your legs straight. Always bend your knees when lifting something, so the bulk of the work is done by the big muscles of your legs, not the small muscles of your lower back. Keep the weight close to your body and your back as straight as possible.

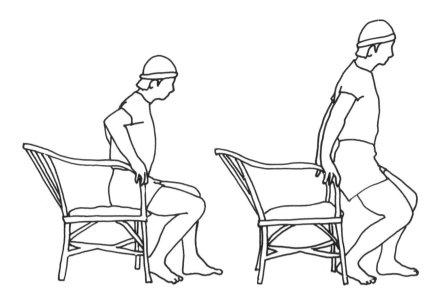

Getting in and out of chairs can be a hazard to your back. Always have one foot in front of the other when rising from a chair. Move your bottom to the edge and, with your back vertical and chin in, use your thigh muscles and arms to push yourself straight up.

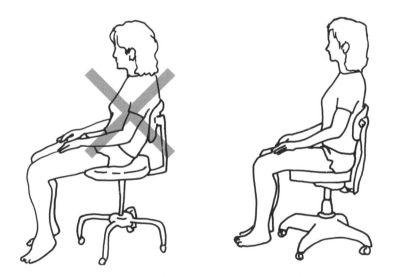

If your shoulders are rounded and your head tends to droop forward, bring yourself into new alignment. This position, when practiced regularly, will lessen back tension and keep the body fresh with energy. Pull your chin in slightly (not down, not up), with the back of your head being pulled straight up. Think of your shoulders being down. Breathe with the idea that you want the middle of your back to expand outward. Tighten your abdominal muscles as you flatten your lower back into the chair. Do this while driving or sitting to take pressure off the lower back. Practice this often and you will naturally train your muscles to hold this more alive alignment without conscious effort.

If you stand in one place for a period of time, as when doing the dishes, prop one foot up on a box or short stool. This will relieve some of the back tension that comes from prolonged standing.

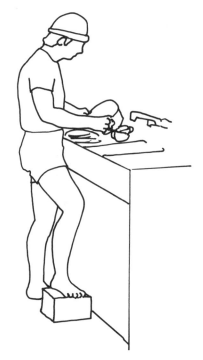

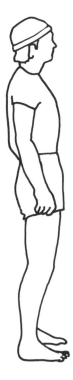

When standing, your knees should be slightly bent (½ inch), with feet pointed straight ahead. Keeping the knees slightly bent prevents the hips from rotating forward. Use the big muscles in the front of the upper legs *(quadriceps)* to control your posture when standing.

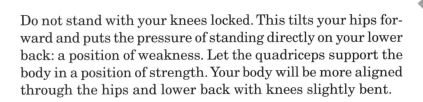

Do not stand with your knees locked. This tilts your hips forward and puts the pressure of standing directly on your lower back: a position of weakness. Let the quadriceps support the body in a position of strength. Your body will be more aligned through the hips and lower back with knees slightly bent.

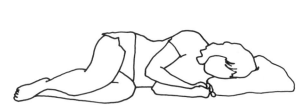

A good, firm sleeping surface helps in back care. If possible, sleep on one side or the other. Sleeping on your stomach can cause tightness in the lower back. If you sleep on your back, a pillow under your knees will keep your lower back flat and minimize tension.

When you are aware that your posture is bad, automatically adjust into a more upright, energetic position. Good posture is developed through the constant awareness of how you sit, stand, walk, and sleep.

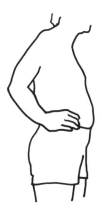

Many tight and so-called bad backs can be caused by excessive weight around the middle. Without the support of strong abdominal muscles, this extra weight will gradually cause a forward pelvic tilt, causing pain and tension in the lower back.

1. Develop the abdominal muscles by regularly doing abdominal curls. Exercise within your limits. It takes time and regularity. But if you don't get into it, the condition will only worsen.

2. Develop the muscles of the chest and arms by doing knee push-ups. These push-ups isolate the muscles in the upper body without straining the lower back. Start an easy three-set routine such as 10–8–6, or whatever —just get started!

3. Stretch the muscles in the front of each hip as shown on p. 51, and stretch the muscles of the lower back *(pp. 26–33 and 63–67)*. By strengthening the abdominal area and stretching the hip and back areas, you can gradually undo the forward pelvic tilt that is, in so many cases, the main cause of back problems.

4. Slowly let the size of your stomach shrink by not overeating.

5. Learn how to walk before you jog, and jog before you run. If you walk a mile a day (at one time) every day, without increasing your calorie intake, you will lose ten pounds of fat in one year.

PNF Stretching

PNF is the abbreviation for "proprioceptive neuromuscular facilitation," a physical therapy developed after World War II to help rehabilitate soldiers suffering from neurological disorders. By the '60s and '70s, physical therapists and sports trainers began using PNF techniques to increase flexibility and range of motion for healthy people, including athletes. In ensuing years, PNF practices have gained popularity with trainers and athletes seeking to optimize sports performance.

Though this book is primarily about static stretching, I have also included some basic PNF stretches. PNF is most often used by athletes and by individuals who have less-than-normal range of motion or who have lost normal range of motion. The PNF stretches in this book can be done without a partner or assisting device. They are easy to learn and use. These stretches are mainly the *contract-relax technique* and the *antagonist contract-relax technique*. Following are descriptions and examples of these two types of PNF stretches.

Contract-Relax-Stretch Technique

Here the muscle is passively taken through a range of motion that produces a mild (not painful) stretch tension, then contracted (as forceful as a closed fist) for 4–5 seconds, then relaxed momentarily, and then taken once again into a mild static stretch for 5–15 seconds. This process may be repeated several times. Each time you can expect a slight increase in tension-free flexibility.

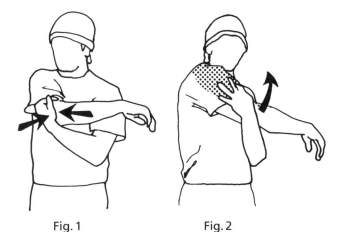

Fig. 1   Fig. 2

Isometric contraction—a muscular contraction in which you increase muscle tension, but the muscles do not lengthen and the joints do not move.

Important: Because of the moderate isometric contraction required in PNF, individuals with heart disease or high blood pressure should be cautioned in the use of PNF. (My approach to isometric contractions is to exert much less than maximal effort.)

Pull your elbow across your chest until a mild (not painful) stretch is felt, then move your elbow away from your body against the resistance of your opposite hand. Now hold a sustained (50–60 percent) isometric contraction for 4–5 seconds *(fig. 1)*. (Do not hold your breath; breathe during contraction of the muscle you will be stretching next.) Relax momentarily and then use your hand and arm to pull your elbow further back across your chest until a mild stretch tension is again felt in the muscles just contracted *(fig. 2)*. Hold a mild (moderate) stretch for 5–15 seconds. Repeat several times.

Antagonist Contract-Relax Technique

The second PNF technique uses the principle of contracting and relaxing opposing muscles, such as with the quadriceps (front thigh) and the hamstrings (back of thigh). In this PNF technique, you contract your quadriceps to relax your hamstrings, then stretch your hamstrings, as in figure 1 or 4. This action facilitates the hamstrings' relaxation through the reciprocal inhibition reflex. (Sounds complicated but is easy to do.) When you contract your quadriceps, as in figure 3, your hamstrings will relax.

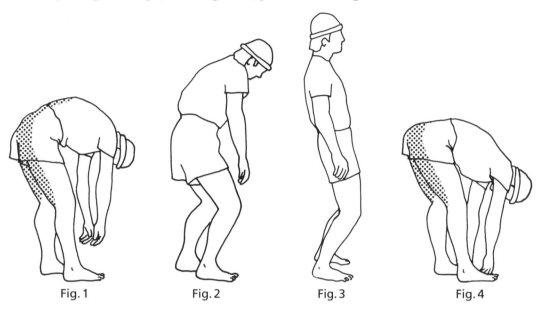

| Fig. 1 | Fig. 2 | Fig. 3 | Fig. 4 |

Try it out. Start in a standing position and slowly bend forward from the hips (keeping knees slightly flexed), until you reach a comfortable stretch (fig. 1). At this time note how far you are able to go. Return to a standing position, keeping your knees slightly flexed as you do so (fig. 2).

Now assume a flexed-knee position, with feet flat and pointed straight ahead (fig. 3). Hold for 15–20 seconds. This position contracts your quadriceps and relaxes your hamstrings, which should make it easier to stretch your hamstrings in the next position. Stand up straight and without bouncing go into the first stretch (fig. 1). Hold for 5–15 seconds or so. You will probably be able to stretch farther now than you could the first time with the same amount of effort. Repeat figures 3 and 1 several times and expect slight-to-moderate flexibility gains (fig. 4).

These two examples should help you to understand and be able to use some basic PNF stretches. The PNF stretches are scattered throughout the book; being mixed in with the sustained (static) stretches. I think the combination of sustained (static) stretches and PNF stretches works quite well.

Caution: Do not overdo the PNF stretches. Stay relaxed and don't strain during mild contractions. Keep breathing! Be comfortable in your approach. Straining and overdoing only leads to not doing!

On the next two pages is a summary of PNF stretches that appear in various places throughout the book.

PNF Stretches

Here are some PNF stretches, as described in the preceding two pages. Try them out to see if the technique works for you (helps you get more flexible). Once you get the idea, you can use the technique on any stretch. Contract-relax-stretch, contract-relax-stretch, etc.

> Repeat each of these series several times. Hold each contraction 4–5 seconds, each stretch 5–15 seconds.

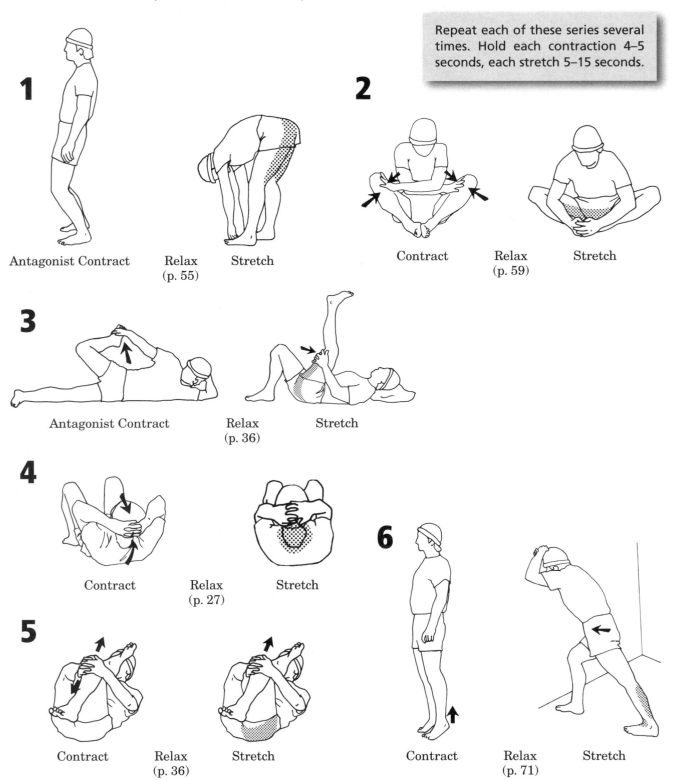

1
Antagonist Contract   Relax (p. 55)   Stretch

2
Contract   Relax (p. 59)   Stretch

3
Antagonist Contract   Relax (p. 36)   Stretch

4
Contract   Relax (p. 27)   Stretch

5
Contract   Relax (p. 36)   Stretch

6
Contract   Relax (p. 71)   Stretch

7

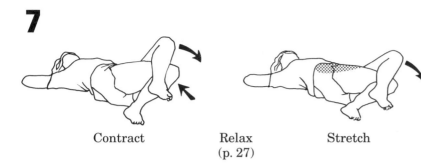

Contract   Relax   Stretch
           (p. 27)

> Don't push it! No pain! *Feel* the stretch.
> Listen to your body.

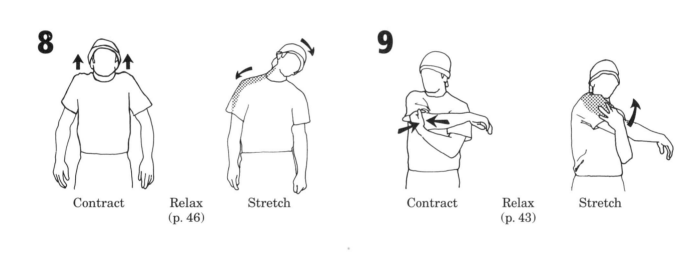

8

Contract   Relax   Stretch
       (p. 46)

9

Contract   Relax   Stretch
       (p. 43)

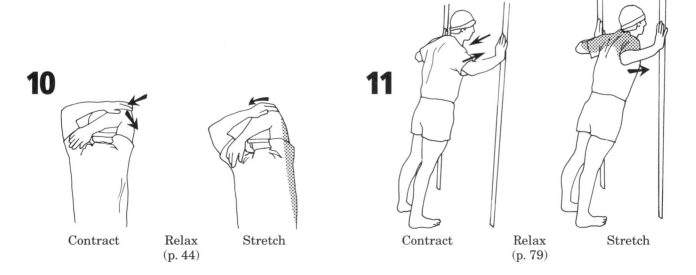

10

Contract   Relax   Stretch
       (p. 44)

11

Contract   Relax   Stretch
       (p. 79)

Body Tools

Body tools are self-help devices that allow you to do body work (massage, acupressure) in a very precise way without a partner. I started using various body tools in the early '90s and found them really helpful. I also discovered that they worked exceptionally well when combined with regular stretching. So I introduced them to the participants at the camps I attended and clinics I gave and the response was excellent.

People like the fact that the tools are easy to use and that they are helpful with trigger points (knotted muscle tissue) and tension. They allow you to work on your body in completely different ways. You can easily access trigger points and sore spots. Tight muscle tissue can be loosened in just a few minutes with most of these tools. They make bodywork easy to do and pain reduction a reality.

Here are some tools that I use regularly and recommend.

TheraCane®

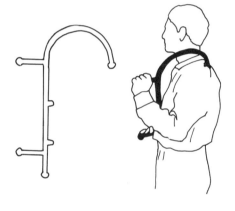

An acupressure tool that loosens tight, painful muscular areas. You use leverage and a slight downward pull to create the desired pressure wherever you want (mild pressure is recommended). Especially designed for the back of the neck, excellent for the mid-back (between shoulder blades), upper back, sides of neck, and shoulders. In fact, it can be used all over the body and even as a stretching aid. This tool has been extremely popular in many pain clinics throughout the United States. It's a great tool that many people find useful.

The Stick®

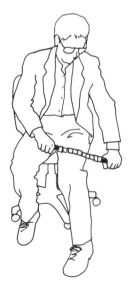

A non-motorized massage device used by serious athletes to loosen "barrier trigger points" (knotted-up muscles). The flexible core with revolving spindles easily molds to various body contours. This tool is wonderful for the legs, especially the calves, and can be used on all major muscle groups. You can use it through clothing or directly on the skin. The Intracell provides instant myofascial release by relaxing healthy muscle fibers and promoting good circulation. Adequate blood supply allows muscles to feel better, work harder, last longer, and recover faster. Using this tool gets the muscles ready for activity, helps disperse lactic acid after a hard workout, helps prevent injuries, and hastens recovery time if injured. I carry one in my CamelBak® water pack on long mountain bike rides and use it along with stretching during resting or eating breaks. It's helpful on that long workout and easy to use.

The Massage Stone®

The Massage Stone is designed with the professional massage therapist in mind. It was designed to aid the hands, not replace them. It's easy to use and is fantastic for self-massage. Because the stone glides over clothing, it can be used often—since you don't have to remove any clothing when you use it. On bare skin it is best to use oils, lotions, or powders so the stone moves smoothly for a natural, soothing effect. Excellent for couples who massage each other; it prevents fingers, thumbs, and wrists from getting sore.

When heated, the Massage Stone drives the heat deep into the muscle tissues, relaxing the muscles for deeper massage. When chilled, the stone can help reduce the inflammation of a sports injury. Just 30 seconds in cold water chills it quickly and evenly. It really feels great.

Because of its unique design, it can be used from head to toes for gentle, relaxing massage and/or for direct pressure work. Each one is hand-carved and currently available in jade, travertine, black marble, white marble, and other stones.

The Trigger Wheel®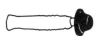

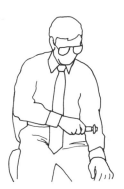

A 2″ nylon wheel on a 4″ handle for deep massage. The Trigger Wheel works on trigger points (knotted muscles) and can be used directly on skin or through light clothing. It works the way a tire rolls back and forth on pavement. Very effective in reaching specific sore spots, such as small areas in the neck, hands, wrists, arms, legs, and feet. You can carry it with you and use it spontaneously throughout the day to keep pain at a minimum.

The Knobble®

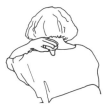

A small, light hand tool for doing deep tissue massage or pressure point release. Saves wear and tear on your hands. Made of solid maple and is easy to carry with you anywhere.

The Foot Massage®

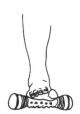

A 2″×9″ roller with raised knobs for foot massage, and rubber rings to protect the floor. A super tool for tired feet. The studded knobs give you pinpoint access to the bottom of the foot. Used to stimulate nerve endings, reduce discomfort, and improve circulation. Use on the job if you sit a lot.

Chinese Reflex Balls

Exercise your hands by rotating the balls in one direction, then the opposite direction. This develops the small muscles of the hands, and improves arm circulation and hand coordination. It also activates acupressure points in the hands. Learn to spin the balls without their touching each other. It takes a little practice, but it's worth it.

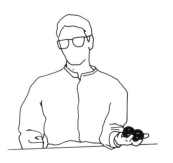

Breath Builder®

This device was originally designed for musicians to develop breath control; however it is excellent for anyone who wishes to develop restorative deep breathing. You blow into a tube and the pressure of your breath keeps a ping-pong ball afloat in the cylinder. It forces you to use your diaphragm muscles and to breathe correctly, with the goal of increasing your lung capacity. Taking more air into your lungs replenishes your bloodstream with oxygen and revitalizes every cell in your body (think of it!). The ball is a visual aid and tells you exactly what your diaphragm is doing by how high the ball floats in the cylinder. Comes with detailed instructions.

The Back Revolution®

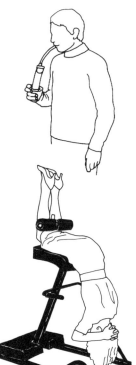

This is a much better tool for inversion than hanging by your feet and ankles. Inverting in this device (with your pelvis stabilized) decompresses discs and works wonders for sore, stiff necks. Health professionals recommend using it for 1 to 3 minutes, 2 to 3 times a day. Also excellent for doing important muscle strengthening back extensions. The easiest way in the world to invert yourself, the device has helped many people control persistent back and neck pain incurred in both industry and professional sports. When I'm home I use it every day.

The Pain Eraser 1®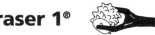

An exceptional hand-held tool that is firm enough for deep massage and yet soft enough for the most tender parts of your body, including your face. Access arms, legs, hands, feet, back, etc. easily with this high quality massage tool. 1½"-wide roller is made of 100% natural rubber with 36 "fingers."

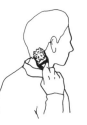

Panasonic Reach Easy®

A gentle multi-surfaced rechargeable massager, perfect for people who want gentle, but effective relief from muscle tension with cordless convenience.

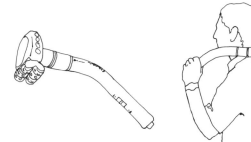

See p. 219 for information on ordering any of these tools.

Recommended Reading

The Alexander Technique: How to Use Your Body without Stress. Wilfred Barlow and Nikolaas Tinbergen. Inner Traditions, Int'l, Richester, Va. 1991.

An updated edition of the classic guide to F. M. Alexander's technique for successful body dynamics.

Awareness through Movement. Moshe Feldenkrais. Harper, San Francisco. 1991.

Illustrated, easy-to-use exercises to improve posture, vision, motivation, and self-awareness.

Beyond Stretching: Russian Flexibility Breakthroughs. Pavel Tsatsouline. Dragon Door Publications, Inc., St. Paul, Minn. 1998.

Are you ready for Pavel? This is a tough, strenuous, take-no-prisoners approach to flexibility and strength. He describes some pretty radical Russian techniques for flexibility, strength, circulation, and healthy joints. Not for wimps; expensive for a paperback.

The Courage to Start: A Guide to Running for Your Life. John "The Penguin" Bingham. Simon & Schuster, New York. 1999.

An inspiring look at the struggles of a man in his 40s learning to run. Funny, witty, and compassionate. Great inspiration for anyone who wants to start running.

Dr. Art Ulene's Complete Guide to Vitamins, Minerals and Herbs. Art Ulene, M.D. Avery Publishing Group, New York. 1999.

Up-to-date info on using increased levels of vitamins, minerals, and herbs to slow the physical deterioration caused by aging.

Galloway's Book on Running. Jeff Galloway. Shelter Publications, Bolinas, Calif. 2002.

This classic has helped many thousands of runners get started and train sensibly. It continues to be a best seller.

Getting in Shape. Bob Anderson, Ed Burke and Bill Pearl. Shelter Publications, Bolinas, Calif. 2002.

How to get back into shape. 30 programs, each with the 3 components of fitness: stretching, weight training, and moving exercises. A simple, visual approach to life-long fitness.

Getting Stronger: Weight Training for Men and Women. Bill Pearl. Shelter Publications, Bolinas, Calif. 2001.

Over half a million copies in print, this is 3 books in one: weight training for sports; bodybuilding; and general conditioning. The most complete book on weight training ever produced.

Healing Moves: How to Cure, Relieve and Prevent Common Ailments with Exercise. Carol Krucoff and Mitchell Krucoff, M.D. Harmony Books, N.Y. 2000.

A timely book by an award-winning health columnist and a renowned cardiologist on the importance of vigorous exercise for general good health. Exercise relieves stress, keeps weight down, improves sleep and helps the body resist illness. There are exercise programs for general health and fitness, as well as exercise prescriptions for specific illnesses and health problems.

Myofascial Pain and Dysfunction, The Trigger Point Manual, Vol 1, Upper Half of Body; Vol 2, The Lower Extremities. Williams and Wilkins, Media, N.Y. 1999.

A classic. Beautifully illustrated. In-depth descriptions and solutions to myofascial pain and dysfunction through trigger point therapy. A reference book that is a pleasure to read and learn from.

Optimal Muscle Recovery for Endurance. Edmund R. Burke, Ph.D. Human Kinetics, Champaign, Ill. 1999.

An excellent guide on how to enhance your recovery, improve performance, and generally feel better. The importance of nutrition, fluid replacement, rest, and body work. A *really* break-through work!

Orthopaedic Sports Medicine: Principles and Practices. Jesse C. DeLee, M.D. and David Drez, Jr., M.D. W. B. Saunders Company, Philadelphia. 1994.

Experts in orthopaedic sports medicine share their experiences in dealing with sports injuries. The contributors give an excellent review of their topic, followed by their recommendations for treatment and recovery. These are not books for casual reading; the 2 volumes are over $250.

Running Within: A Guide to Mastering the Body-Mind-Spirit Connection for Ultimate Training and Racing. Jerry Lynch and Warren A. Scott. Human Kinetics, Champaign, Ill. 1999.

Dr. Lynch brings us to the forefront of sports psychology. Here are mental tools for running farther and faster, as well as for integrating body, mind, and spirit.

Science of Stretching. Michael J. Alter. Human Kinetics, Champaign, Ill. 1999.

A very thorough and technical book on all aspects of flexibility and stretching.

8 Weeks to Optimum Health. Andrew Weil, M.D. Fawcett Books, N.Y. 1998.

Dr. Weil believes in the body's natural abilities to heal. His changes are not radical but rather a series of simple, small steps to optimum health: taking supplements, adjusting eating habits, eliminating toxins from the diet, and an exercise program based on walking and improving breathing patterns.

Super Power Breathing: For Super Energy, High Health & Longevity. Paul C. Bragg and Patricia N. D. Bragg, Ph.D. Health Science, Goleta, Calif. 1999.

Excellent book on using your lungs to improve your health and increase your resistance to disease. A classic.

Touch for Health: A Practical Guide to Natural Health Using Acupressure Touch and Massage. John F. Thie. Devorss & Company, Marina del Rey, Calif. 1979.

How to utilize acupressure effectively, how to use kinesiology to test you body's need for foods, how to guide your own physical well-being. A complete system for home health.

Stretching in the Office. Bob Anderson and Jean Anderson. Shelter Publications, Bolinas, Calif. 2002.

Stretches and exercises for people who work in offices or at computers. Routines that will relieve stress and tension and keep the body tuned. Keep in your desk drawer.

Stretching Prescriptions

Here is a summary of the stretches in this book that can be used by health care professionals when prescribing individual fitness and rehabilitation programs. Circle the stretches that are appropriate for the individual.

Relaxing Stretches for Your Back • *26–33*

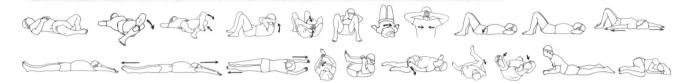

Stretches for the Legs, Feet, and Ankles • *34–41*

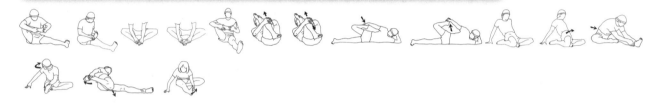

Stretches for the Back, Shoulders, and Arms • *42–48*

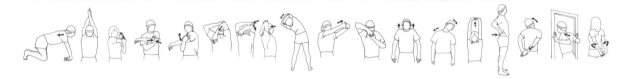

A Series of Stretches for the Legs • *49–53*

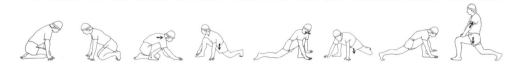

Stretches for the Lower Back, Hips, Groin, and Hamstrings • *54–61*

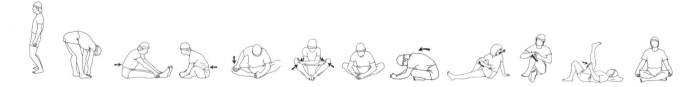

Stretches for the Back, Hips, and Legs • *63–67*

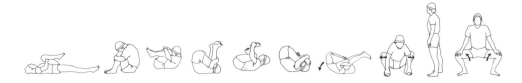

Elevating Your Feet • *68–70*

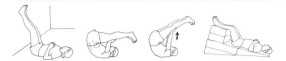

Standing Stretches for the Legs and Hips • *71–77*

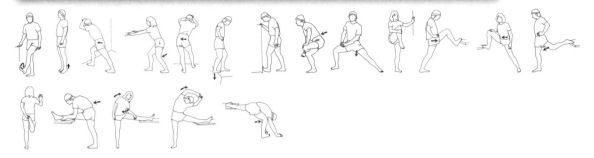

Standing Stretches for the Upper Body • *79–84*

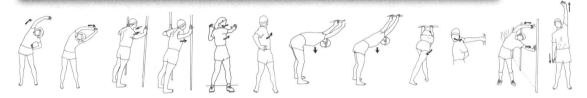

Chin Bar *85* | Upper Body with Towel *86–87* | Stretches for the Hands, Wrists, and Forearms • *88–89*

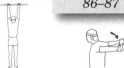

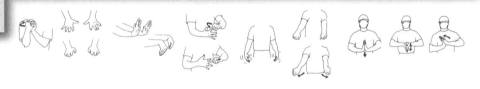

Sitting Stretches • *90–93*

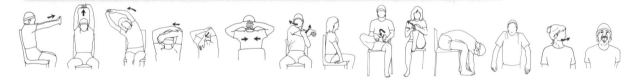

Leg and Groin Stretches with Feet Elevated • *94–96*

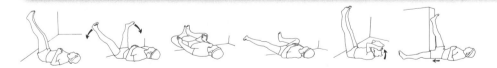

Stretching the Groin and Hips with Feet Apart • *97–100*

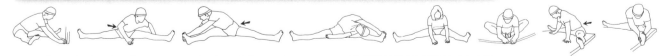

Learning the Splits • *101–102*

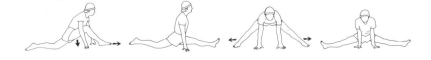

Index

More on Stretching
from Bob and Jean Anderson

Over the past 25 years, Bob and Jean have developed a variety of their own stretching and fitness products, all designed to help people stay flexible and fit. In addition, Bob has discovered a number of body tools and workout products that are distributed by Stretching, Inc.

Stretching Video & DVD

A 57-minute video or DVD organized in six comfortably paced sections: a brief introduction, stretches for the neck and back, then legs and hips, then feet, and finally, the arms and shoulders. The tape and DVD conclude with a 14-minute stretching routine for all body parts that can be used for everyday fitness or for sports. Suitable for people of all ages and interests. (*The DVD is in spoken English and Spanish.*)

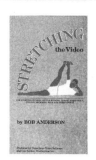

Stretching Charts

These large wall charts are great for learning how to stretch. They not only remind you to stretch (by being so visible), but guide you through a series of stretches (without having to look at the book). They come in both plain paper and laminated, and cover most of the routines in pp. 105–108 in this book.

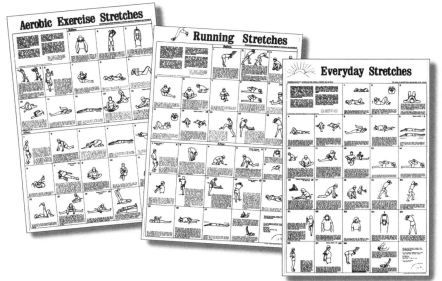

Stretching Chart Pads

These are miniature versions of the wall charts. They measure 8½ by 11 inches and come in pads of 40 identical sheets. As with the wall charts, full instructions are below each stretch. Used frequently by medical professionals, trainers, body workers, and coaches for their clients or team members.

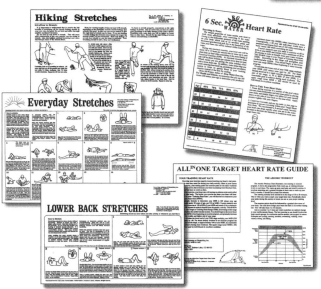

Stretch & Strengthen

This is a spiral-bound book for people in wheelchairs, the disabled, and the elderly. It contains stretching exercises and muscle-strengthening exercises performed with a circular resistive cord with tubular handles. Valuable for rehabilitation and for disabled people who want to increase their strength and flexibility.

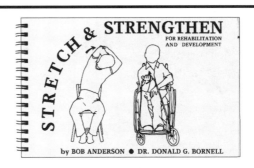

Body Tools

Body tools can be used in conjunction with stretching to help reduce muscular tension and pain. *(See pp. 210–212.)*

Shown here are: (1) TheraCane® (2) Pain Eraser 2® (3) Knobble® (4) Pain Eraser 1® (5) The Foot Massage® (6) Ancient Oil® (7) Panasonic Reach Easy® (8) Trigger Wheel® (9) Breath Builder® (10) Chinese Reflex Balls (11) Massage Stone® (12) The Stick®.

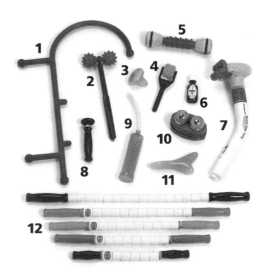

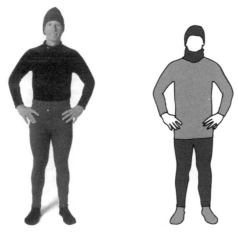

Maxit® Workout Gear

Functional sportswear for the person who wants warmth and dryness (97 percent wind-resistant) and breathability without layering. Not high fashion (no neon colors or billboard look), but this blend of spun polyolefin (a new generation of polypropelene) and Lycra® is comfortable and durable. This is the clothing many NFL players wear under their uniforms in cold-weather games. Great for all cold climate activities.

The Back Revolution®

An inversion support system for true spinal decompression and muscular strengthening of the back, abdominal, and oblique regions of the body. This very stable gravity traction machine supports you so you are inverted from the hips and upper thigh area, not your ankles. Being inverted for a minimum of 70 seconds decompresses your spine, relieves lower back pain, and stretches your back and abdominal muscles.

Call 1-800-333-1307 for a free color catalog or visit Stretching's website at **www.stretching.com**

More World-Class Fitness Books from Shelter Publications

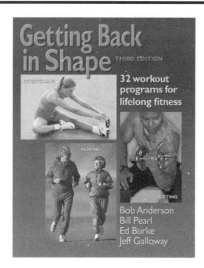

Getting Back in Shape
32 *Workout Programs for Lifelong Fitness*
Bob Anderson, Bill Pearl, Ed Burke, and Jeff Galloway
Illustrated by Jean Anderson

A unique workout book for anyone who wants to get back in shape.

- Stretching, weightlifting, and cardiovascular training
- Three-point programs
- "Simple programs designed for the busy schedule."
  —*Kiplinger's Personal Finance* magazine

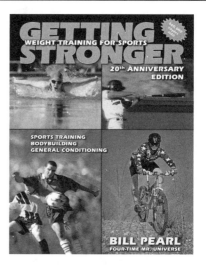

Getting Stronger, 20th Anniversary Edition
Weight Training for Sports
Bill Pearl

A revised edition of the best-seller on weight training. Of special interest to runners are off-season and in-season weight training programs for distance running and new rehab exercises for knees.

- 550,000 copies sold
- 80 one-page training programs
- General conditioning, sports training, and bodybuilding
- "A must for anyone serious about fitness."
  —*Newsday*

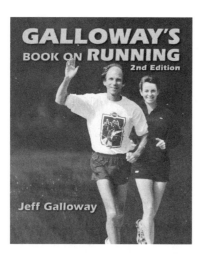

Galloway's Book on Running, 2nd Edition
Jeff Galloway

A complete revision of Olympian Jeff Galloway's classic book on running

- 430,000 copies of original edition sold
- Training programs for 5K, 10K, and half-marathons
- The second running boom
- New info on diet, slow running, clothing, and shoes

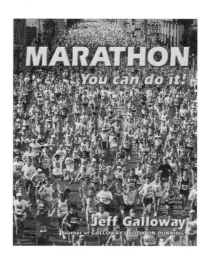

Marathon
You Can Do It!
Jeff Galloway

A revolutionary new book on marathon training

"Provides the inspiration to make almost anyone want to run a marathon, and enough training and racing strategies to guarantee that everyone who tries it will succeed."

–Amby Burfoot, Editor, *Runner's World*

Stay Fit in the Office

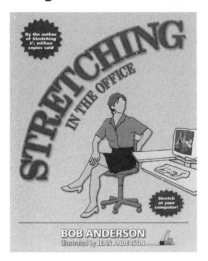

Stretching in the Office

Bob Anderson
Illustrated by Jean Anderson

A solution to the hidden health crisis in the high-tech workplace, this book shows you how to stay pain-free and flexible while spending long hours each day at a computer or desk. There are hundreds of drawings and 20 illustrated stretching routines you can do while at the computer, sitting for long periods, or talking on the phone.

• "The stretches will ward off repetitive stress injuries, soothe back and neck pain, and simply buffer the effects of a bad day."

—*Kiplinger's Personal Finance magazine*

Visit our online Office Fitness Clinic for stretching routines you can print out and use in the office.

www.shelterpub.com

Software that Reminds You to Stretch

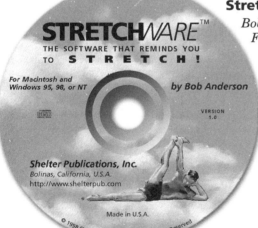

StretchWare™

Bob Anderson
For Macintosh (OS X and Classic) and
Windows 95 / 98 / ME / 2000 / NT / XP / Vista

The machine that causes the problem now contains the solution!

This new computer program is based on the book, *Stretching in the Office*.

• Periodically, your computer asks if you want to stretch.
• If you say yes, the stretches appear on screen.
• When you roll your mouse over a stretch, instructions for that stretch pop up in a small window.
• You set your own preferences as to timing, types of stretches, sounds, etc.

"An electronic tap-on-the-shoulder."

—*San Jose Mercury News*

"A great program, ingeniously simple, yet highly effective. It works seamlessly with other software. . . ."

—*PA Today*

Test Drive StretchWare™!
Download a fully-functioning version that you can try out for 30 days.

www.stretchware.com

Shelter Publications
P.O. Box 279
Bolinas, CA 94924
415-868-0280
800-307-0131 (orders)

About the Authors

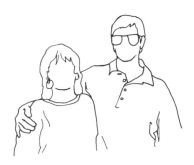

Bob Anderson is the world's most popular stretching authority. For over 25 years, Bob has taught millions of people his simple approach to stretching.

Bob and his wife Jean first published a home-made version of *Stretching* in a garage in southern California in 1975. The drawings were done by Jean, based on photos she took of Bob doing the stretches. This book was modified and published by Shelter Publications in 1980 for general bookstore distribution and is now known by lay people as well as medical professionals as the most user-friendly book on the subject. To date it has sold over 3 million copies worldwide and has been translated into 19 languages.

Bob is fit and healthy these days, but it wasn't always so. In 1968, he was overweight (190 pounds—at 5′9″) and out of shape. He began a personal fitness program that got him down to 135 pounds. Yet one day, while in a physical conditioning class in college, he found he couldn't reach much past his knees in a straight-legged sitting position. So Bob started stretching. He found he soon felt better and that stretching made his running and cycling easier.

The American fitness boom was just starting, and the millions of people who started working out were discovering the importance of flexibility in their fitness programs. After several years of exercising and stretching with Jean and a small group of friends, Bob gradually developed a method of stretching that could be taught to anyone. Soon he was teaching his technique to others.

He began with professional sports teams: the Denver Broncos, the California (now Anaheim) Angels, the Los Angeles Dodgers, the Los Angeles Lakers, and the New York Jets. He also worked with college teams at Nebraska, UC Berkeley, Washington State, and Southern Methodist University, as well as other amateur and Olympic athletes in a variety of sports. He traveled around the country for years, teaching stretching to people at sports medicine clinics, athletic clubs, and running camps.

Since then, Bob continues to teach at running camps (Jeff Galloway's in particular), cycling camps, medical ski seminars, and at Jimmy Heuga's clinics for people with multiple sclerosis.

In the 1980s, Bob was a serious mountain runner and road biker. For ten years in a row he ran the Catalina Island Marathon in southern California, the 18-mile Imogen Pass run in Telluride, Colorado (which goes up over a 13,000-foot-high ridge), and the Pike's Peak Marathon. These days Bob spends most of his workout time on a mountain bike and running in the mountains above his house in Colorado, often going for 3–5 hour bike rides in the mountains, with occasional trips to Utah. Though Bob works out a lot, he knows that training like this is not necessary for the average person to be fit. Through his travels, lectures, and workshops, he's kept in constant touch with people in all degrees of physical condition.

Jean Anderson has a B.A. in art from California State University at Long Beach. She began running and cycling (and stretching) with Bob in 1970. She developed a system of shooting photos of Bob doing the stretches, then making clear ink drawings of each stretch position. Jean was photographer, illustrator, typesetter, and editor of the first homemade edition of *Stretching*. These days she oversees Stretching Inc.'s mail-order business and hikes, cycles, and plays tennis to stay in shape.

Credits

Editor
Lloyd Kahn

Production Manager
Rick Gordon

Design
Rick Gordon, Lloyd Kahn, Jean Anderson

Graphics Production
Robert Lewandowski

Design Consultation
David Wills

Proofreading & Indexing
Frances Bowles

Models
Bob Anderson
Jean Anderson
Tiffany Anderson
Shari Boesel
Paul Comish
Kim Cooper
Debra Gentile
Karen Johnston
Bob Kahn
Will Kahn
Jim Melo
Justine Melo
Victoria Pollard
Christina Reski
Dave Roche
JoAnne Sercl
Kelsey Sercl
Shane Sercl
Mary Ann Shipstad
Shawntel Staab
Peggy Sterling
Joyce Werth

Production Hardware
Apple Macintosh G3/400, Power Computing
PowerCenter Pro 210, Agfa Arcus II scanner,
GCC Elite XL 20/600 laser printer,
Epson Stylus Color 3000 printer

Production Software
QuarkXPress, Adobe Photoshop, Microsoft
Word, Nisus Writer

Typefaces
New Century Schoolbook, Frutiger

Printing
Malloy, Inc., Ann Arbor, Michigan, U.S.A.

Paper
60 lb. Glatfelter Thor Plus D-56 paper

Special thanks to the following people,
who helped with this book in one way or
another:

Joan Creed
Drake Jordan
Lesley Kahn
The folks at Publishers Group West
Brian Roberts
George Young